ARE YOU SAFE?
PHARMACOVIGILANCE

Rajesh Kumar Mukherjee,
Dilip Kumar Roy.

Content

parameters

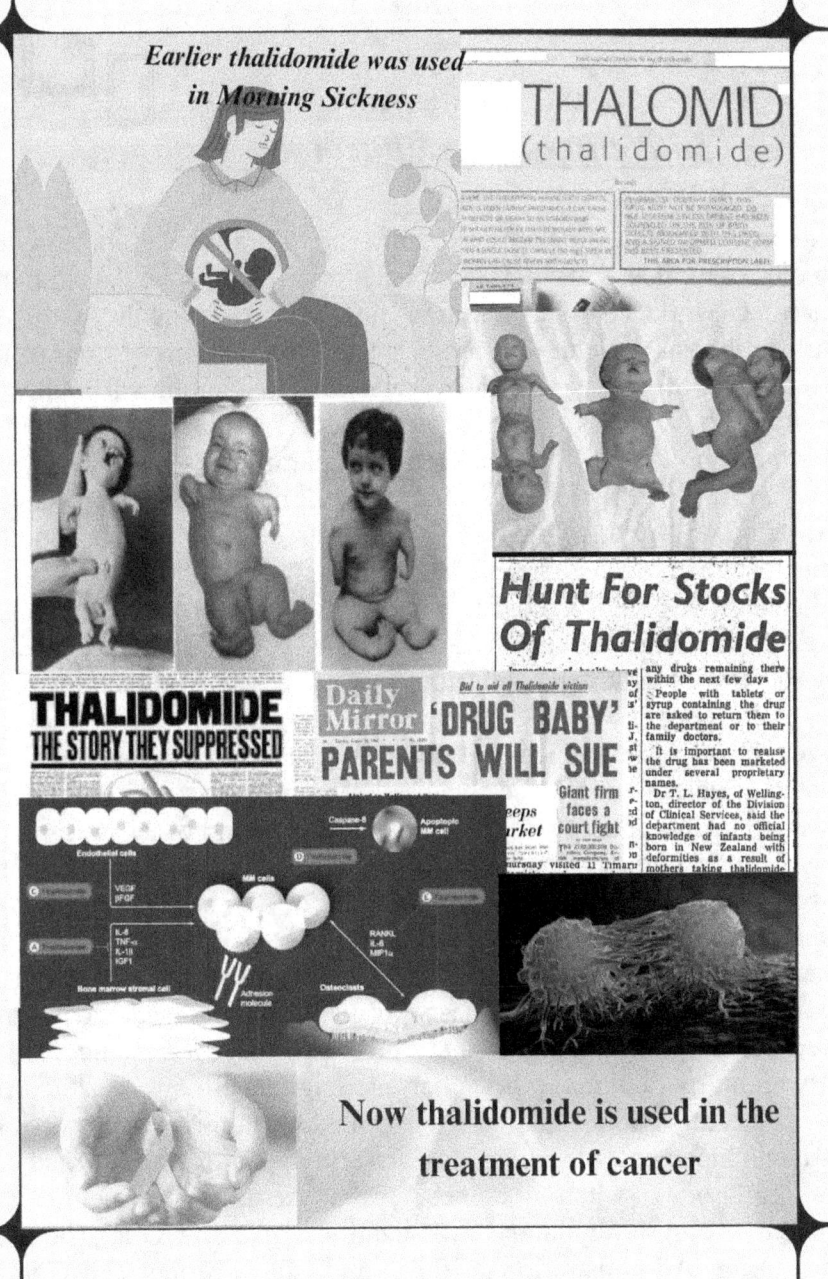

Earlier thalidomide was used in Morning Sickness

Now thalidomide is used in the treatment of cancer

Unit 1

Chapter 1
Introduction to Pharmacovigilance

The process of keeping an eye on the safety of medications and other medical supplies after they have been approved for use is known as pharmacovigilance. It's a scientific field that deals with data collection, assessment, detection, monitoring, and prevention of side effects and other drug-related issues. The foundation of medication safety and a vital component of every healthcare system is pharmacovigilance. Its objective is to guarantee the safest and most efficient use of medications. Pharmacovigilance includes tasks like gathering, evaluating, and disclosing adverse drug reactions; spotting drug usage trends; and giving medical professionals input on the efficacy and safety of medications. It may also involve keeping an eye out for drug interactions, analyzing how well drugs are labelled, and determining how prescription drugs affect general health.

Overview of Pharmacovigilance: A vital part of the healthcare system, pharmacovigilance focuses on the identification, evaluation, comprehension, and avoidance of side effects and other drug-related issues. The Greek terms "pharmakon," which means drug, and "vigilare," which means to keep watch, are the source of the name "pharmacovigilance", it's main objectives are to guarantee pharmaceutical products' safety and to assist in the comprehensive benefit-risk assessment of these products over the course of their lifecycle. By confirming that the advantages of medications outweigh any potential risks, pharmacovigilance plays a critical role in preserving public health. It supports the continuous assessment and enhancement of medication safety and aids in the decision-making process when it comes to the use of pharmaceuticals in clinical settings. regulatory organizations, like the U.S. The Food and Drug Administration (FDA) and the European Medicines Agency (EMA), which also establishes guidelines for their execution, supervise pharmacovigilance efforts.

Among the duties of pharmacovigilance are:

1. Monitoring adverse drug reactions (ADRs) involves identifying and gathering data on unfavorable occurrences or reactions associated with medication usage, as well as reporting and recording ADRs by patients, healthcare providers, and pharmaceutical corporations.

2. Signal detection is the methodical examination of data to find possible signals or patterns that might point to hazards or safety issues with a given medication that have not yet been identified.

3. Risk assessment is the process of analyzing the frequency and severity of adverse events to ascertain how they affect a drug's benefit-risk profile.

4. Risk management is the application of tactics to reduce or manage hazards that have been discovered, such as creating and disseminating safety information to the public and medical professionals.

5. Regulatory Compliance: Ensuring that the safety monitoring of medications complies with regulatory regulations; this may include sending safety reports to health authorities on a regular basis.

6. Post-Marketing Surveillance: The ongoing observation of medications following their approval and release to the public, with the possibility that side effects will surface in a wider range of patient populations.

7. Communication and Education: Providing patients, healthcare providers, and the general public with accurate and current information regarding drug safety.

8. Cooperation and Information Sharing: To improve the general awareness of drug safety, cooperation is needed between regulatory bodies, pharmaceutical companies, healthcare providers, and patients.

1.1. The origins and progression of pharmacovigilance:

Pharmacovigilance has a long history and has grown over several decades in response to growing concerns regarding the safety of pharmaceutical products, the following is a timeline of significant turning points in the development of pharmacovigilance:

a. **Thalidomide Tragedy (1950s–1960s):** The thalidomide tragedy, which occurred in the late 1950s and early 1960s and resulted in serious birth deformities in new-borns, brought attention to the necessity of comprehensive drug safety monitoring. Because of this incident, people became more aware of the possible risks associated with pharmaceutical products, which in turn prompted the creation of regulatory frameworks for post-marketing surveillance and drug approval.

b. **WHO Adverse Reaction Monitoring Program (1968):** In 1968, the World Health Organization (WHO) introduced the International Drug Monitoring Program, objective of this vigorous work was to gather and examine data on adverse drug reactions (ADRs) throughout the world, this data is centrally stored at the WHO Collaborating Centre for International Drug Monitoring, which is situated in Uppsala, Sweden.

c. **The 1970s saw the establishment of regulatory agencies—** organizations like the U.S. The European Medicines Agency (EMA) and the Food and Drug Administration (FDA) started integrating pharmacovigilance into their regulatory procedures. To standardize the reporting and evaluation of adverse occurrences, guidelines and standards were created.

d. **Emphasis on Risk Management and Signal Detection (1980s–1990s):** In the 1980s and 1990s, risk management and signal detection received more attention. More people realized how crucial it was to keep an eye on drug safety throughout the whole product lifecycle, even after it was put on the market.

e. **International Conference on Harmonization (ICH):** To standardize regulatory criteria across various locations, the International Conference on Harmonization of Technical Criteria for Registration of Pharmaceuticals for Human Use (ICH) was founded in the 1990s. The ICH guidelines, which encompass pharmacovigilance standards, have been instrumental in bringing about global standardization of processes.

f. **Good Pharmacovigilance Practices (GVP):** Developed in 2012 by the European Medicines Agency (EMA), GVPs offer a complete framework for conducting pharmacovigilance activities inside the European Union. The GVP recommendations address a number of topics, such as safety reporting, signal detection, and risk management.

g. **Information Technology Advancements (21st Century):** The 21st century has seen advances in information technology that have made it possible for pharmacovigilance data to be collected, analyzed, and shared more effectively. The capacity to identify and evaluate medication safety signals has improved thanks to the use of electronic databases, data mining methods, and international communication networks.

h. **Global Pharmacovigilance Network Extension:** Global pharmacovigilance networks and international cooperation are becoming more and more significant. Global regulatory bodies can communicate information and work together more easily thanks to organizations like the WHO, the Council for International Organizations of Medical Sciences (CIOMS), and the Pharmaceutical Inspection Co-operation Scheme (PIC/S), pharmacovigilance is always changing and a continuous efforts are directed toward boosting risk management tactics, guaranteeing a proactive approach to drug safety during the course of pharmaceutical product lifecycles, and increasing the effectiveness of signal detection.

1.2. The significance of medication safety oversight:

Pharmacovigilance the safety monitoring of pharmaceuticals justification crucial for a number of reasons, including patient safety and public health preservation, the following are the main points that highlight how crucial safety monitoring is:

1. Patient safety: Preserving patients' health and wellbeing is the main objective of safety monitoring. Healthcare providers can reduce the risks connected with medication use by recognizing and resolving adverse drug reactions (ADRs) and other safety concerns.

2. Early Adverse Event Detection: Safety monitoring makes it possible to identify unanticipated side effects and adverse events early on that could not have been seen during clinical trials. Healthcare professionals can adjust treatment programs or supply substitute medications when identification occurs in a timely manner.

3. Risk-Benefit Assessment: An ongoing assessment of how well a medication balances its risks and benefits is made possible by ongoing safety monitoring. By ensuring that a drug's therapeutic benefits outweigh any potential side effects, this dynamic assessment helps patients and healthcare providers make well-informed decisions.

4. Protection of Public Health: Keeping an eye on medication safety is essential to broader public health protection. By recognizing and resolving safety issues, we may help stop widespread harm and make sure that the public is only given access to safe and effective pharmaceuticals.

5. Adherence to regulations: Safety monitoring is required by regulatory bodies as part of their supervision of pharmaceutical products. Pharmacovigilance regulations must be followed in order for a drug to be approved and for market authorization to continue. In order to prove the continued safety of their goods, pharmaceutical companies are required to provide safety data and reports to regulatory organizations.

6. Developing trust in healthcare: Patients, healthcare providers, and the general public can all benefit from open and thorough safety monitoring procedures. People are more likely to have faith in the healthcare system when they are assured that the medications they take are regularly inspected for safety.

7. Identification of rare and long-term effects: Certain side effects of medications may be uncommon or develop gradually. Such incidents, which may go unnoticed throughout the comparatively brief course of clinical trials, are captured with the use of safety monitoring, this is especially crucial for drugs used as long-term treatments or for chronic illnesses.

8. Enhancing treatment guidelines and drug labels: Safety monitoring yields important data that can be used to update treatment guidelines and drug labels. New safety information is added to labels to ensure patients and healthcare providers are informed about potential dangers and can use medications appropriately.

9. Post-marketing surveillance: Despite extensive testing before approval, real-world use of medications may uncover new safety issues. Safety monitoring makes post-marketing surveillance possible, which enables ongoing evaluation of a drug's safety profile across a range of patient populations and environments.

1.3. The International Drug Monitoring Program of the World Health Organization:

The International Drug Monitoring Programme is a universal initiative that the World Health Organization (WHO) set in motion in 1968 to monitor and improve the safety of pharmaceuticals. The program's main focus is on gathering and analysing data about adverse drug reactions (ADRs) and other issues pertaining to drugs. The WHO International Drug Monitoring Program has the following main features:

Foundation and Goals: Designed to support global cooperation in tracking and disclosing medication side effects, the program was started in the wake of the thalidomide disaster, the main goals are to encourage the safe and efficient use of medications, share safety information worldwide, and identify adverse drug reactions (ADRs) as soon as possible, WHO Collaborating Centre for International Drug Monitoring was situated at Uppsala, Sweden, the WHO Collaborating Centre for International Drug Monitoring provides support for the program, this center is the global repository for individual case safety reports (ICSRs) that member nations submit, participating nations provide Individual Case Safety Reports (ICSRs), which are comprehensive reports on specific instances of possible adverse medication reactions. These reports provide details on the suspected medication, the patient, and any adverse events that have been documented.

a. Global Database of Individual Case Safety Reports (ICSRs): The WHO Collaborating Center keeps an international database of ICSRs, which makes it possible to compile and analyze safety information from all over the world. The WHO Global Individual Case Safety Report (ICSR) database, also referred to as VigiBase, is this database.

b. VigiBase with signal detection: VigiBase makes signal detection easier. Signal detection is the process of systematically analyzing safety data to find possible signals or trends that could point to hazards related to certain pharmaceuticals that have not yet been identified.

c. International network of pharmacovigilance centers: A network of national pharmacovigilance centers spread across several nations powers the initiative. These centers work together to communicate, analyze, and gather safety-related data.

d. Cooperation with regulatory bodies: To improve the overall safety monitoring of medications, the WHO program works closely with pharmaceutical companies, national regulatory bodies, and other stakeholders.

e. Training and capacity building: By offering technical assistance and training, the initiative helps the pharmacovigilance systems in participating nations grow in strength.

f. Publication of safety information: To inform the international medical community on safety information and discoveries, the WHO Collaborating Center regularly publishes reports and newsletters.

g. Advocacy for Pharmacovigilance: The program offers advice and guidance to enhance the caliber and efficacy of safety monitoring initiatives across the globe, while also promoting the significance of pharmacovigilance.

The WHO International Drug Monitoring Programme has greatly aided international cooperation and communication in the field of pharmacovigilance. The program plays a significant role in the ongoing efforts to improve the safety of medicines globally by facilitating the exchange of safety information and aiding in signal detection.

1.4. India's Pharmacovigilance Program of India

(PvPI): The Ministry of Health & Family Welfare, Government of India, initiated the pharmacovigilance program of India (PvPI) to keep an eye on the safety of medications in the nation. In 2010, PvPI was formally introduced and functions under the Central Drugs Standard Control Organization (CDSCO), India's national pharmaceutical regulatory body. The following are the main aspect of the Indian Pharmacovigilance Program:

Goals: By tracking and assessing adverse drug reactions (ADRs) and other drug-related issues, PvPI seeks to improve patient safety.

The program aims to support international pharmacovigilance initiatives and establish a national database of drug safety data.

National Coordination Center (NCC): The Indian Pharmacopoeia Commission (IPC) in Ghaziabad, Uttar Pradesh, is home to the National Coordination Center for PvPI. The NCC acts as the national center for the coordination of pharmacovigilance initiatives.

The Adverse Drug Reaction Monitoring Centers (AMCs) are a network of facilities that PvPI has set up all over India. These facilities, which are frequently found in hospitals and medical schools, are essential for gathering and disseminating data on negative drug reactions.

Indian Pharmacopoeia Commission (IPC): The IPC is the PvPI secretariat and is essential to the operation of the program. It makes communication easier between AMCs, drug manufacturers, medical professionals, and government regulators.

Pharmacovigilance Data Repository (PvDR): PvPI is responsible for the upkeep of this extensive database, which houses and organizes data on adverse drug reactions that have been reported from a variety of sources.

Partnership with International Organizations and Networks for Global Pharmacovigilance: PvPI works in partnership with global pharmacovigilance initiatives, such as the World Health Organization (WHO) and the Uppsala Monitoring Centre, to exchange resources and knowledge while also making a positive impact on the field.

Training and Capacity Building: For healthcare workers, pharmacists, and other stakeholders engaged in pharmacovigilance activities, PvPI offers training courses and capacity-building programs, pharmaceutical companies must abide by pharmacovigilance regulations and report any negative events to PvPI. Drug approval, marketing authorization, and post-marketing surveillance all depend on compliance.

Public Awareness and Education: To inform patients, healthcare providers, and the general public about the significance of reporting adverse drug reactions, PvPI runs public awareness campaigns. This contributes to a culture of reporting and promotes active participation in pharmacovigilance.

Frequent Reporting and Analysis: PvPI summarizes safety data and analysis in reports and newsletters that are released on a regular basis. These reports provide insights into the safety profiles of drugs in the Indian market, the Pharmacovigilance Program of India plays a critical role in ensuring the safety of medicines used in the country. By fostering collaboration, collecting comprehensive safety data, and promoting awareness, PvPI contributes to the continuous improvement of drug safety standards and practices in India, adverse drug reactions (ADRs) are any harmful or unexpected reactions that occur as a result of taking a drug or a combination of drugs. The most common type of ADR is an allergic reaction, which can range from mild to severe. Other types of ADRs can include gastrointestinal distress, skin reactions, and organ damage. Some ADRs can be life-threatening and may require immediate medical attention.

Chapter 2
Introduction to adverse drug reactions

Adverse drug reactions (ADRs) refer to unintended and harmful effects resulting from the use of medications at normal doses during proper administration. These reactions can occur in response to prescription or over-the-counter drugs, as well as herbal remedies, vitamins, and other supplements. Adverse drug reactions can vary widely in severity, ranging from mild side effects to life-threatening conditions.

Types of adverse drug reactions:

a. Side effects: predictable and often mild reactions that are well-known and documented for a particular drug. They usually occur at therapeutic doses and may include symptoms like drowsiness, nausea, or headaches.

b. Allergic reactions: immune system-mediated responses that can lead to symptoms such as rash, itching, swelling, or, in severe cases, anaphylaxis.

c. Idiosyncratic reactions: Unpredictable and uncommon reactions that are not related to the known pharmacological actions of the drug. Individual genetic factors can have an impact on these reactions.

d. Incidence and prevalence: Adverse drug reactions contribute significantly to hospital admissions, morbidity, and mortality. The incidence varies depending on factors such as patient population, drug characteristics, and prescribing patterns, certain populations such as the elderly and individuals with multiple chronic conditions, may be more susceptible to adverse drug reactions.

e. Risk factors: Patient-related Factors: Age, gender, genetics, pre-existing medical conditions, and individual variations in drug metabolism can influence the likelihood of experiencing an adverse drug reaction.

f. Drug-related factors: Dosage, duration of use, drug interactions, and the specific pharmacological properties of a drug can contribute to the risk of adverse reactions.

g. Monitoring and reporting: Continuous monitoring of patients during drug therapy is essential to detect and manage adverse drug reactions promptly. Healthcare professionals are encouraged to report adverse drug reactions to regulatory authorities, contributing to the ongoing evaluation of a drug's safety profile.

h. Prevention and management: Health professionals play a crucial role in preventing adverse drug reactions through thorough patient assessment, proper drug selection, and monitoring. If an adverse drug reaction occurs, management may involve discontinuing the offending drug, providing supportive care, and, in some cases, administering specific antidotes.

i. Regulatory framework: The regulatory bodies, such as the European Medicines Agency (EMA) and U.S. Food and Drug Administration (FDA) play a vital role in evaluating and monitoring the safety of drugs throughout their lifecycle.

2.1. Definitions and classification of ADRs:

Adverse Drug Reaction (ADR): Definition: Any response to a drug that is noxious and unintended, occurring at doses used for the prevention, diagnosis, or treatment of a medical condition, it can be classified and defined based on various criteria, including their nature, severity, onset, and predictability.

Classification: ADRs are commonly categorized based on their nature, severity, and underlying mechanisms.

Nature of adverse drug reactions includes:

a. Type A (augmented) reactions: predictable and dose-dependent responses that are an extension of the drug's pharmacological effects. Examples include gastrointestinal disturbances or bleeding associated with NSAIDs.

b. Type B (Bizarre) reactions: Unpredictable and not related to the drug's pharmacological actions. These reactions often have an immunological basis and include allergies or idiosyncratic responses.

c. Onset of adverse drug reactions: Immediate Reactions: They occur shortly after drug administration and are often related to immunological mechanisms (e.g., anaphylaxis).

d. Delayed reactions: Manifest days to weeks after drug exposure and may involve immune-mediated processes (e.g., drug-induced liver injury) or delayed hypersensitivity reactions.

Predictability of adverse drug reactions includes:
Type I (predictable) Reactions: dose-dependent and often related to the known pharmacological actions of the drug.
Type II (unpredictable) Reactions: not related to the known pharmacological actions, often idiosyncratic, and less predictable. Examples include hypersensitivity reactions.

Organ system involvement: ADRs can affect specific organ systems, leading to categories such as dermatological reactions, hematological reactions, cardiovascular reactions, etc.
Dose-response relationship: Some ADRs exhibit a clear relationship to the drug dose, while others do not follow a typical dose-response pattern.
Seriousness and causality assessment: Regulatory agencies often classify ADRs based on their seriousness and likelihood of being causally related to the drug. This includes terms such as "serious," "unexpected," and "suspected."
Common terminology: Side Effects: Unintended, often mild, and expected reactions occurring at therapeutic doses.
Toxic Effects: Dose-dependent reactions resulting from drug accumulation or excessive dosing.
Allergic Reactions: Immunologically mediated responses involving the immune system.

2.2. Detection and reporting: Detecting and reporting adverse drug reactions (ADRs) are crucial steps in ensuring the safety of patients and improving the overall pharmacovigilance of medications.
Detection of adverse drug reactions includes:
   a. **Clinical monitoring:** Healthcare professionals play a key role in detecting ADRs through routine clinical monitoring of patients receiving medications,observing and documenting any unexpected or unusual symptoms or changes in laboratory values.

b. **Patient reporting:** encouraging patients to report any perceived adverse effects or changes in health while taking medications; gathering information about over-the-counter drugs, herbal supplements, and other non-prescription substances.
c. **Laboratory monitoring:** Regular monitoring of relevant laboratory parameters to detect potential ADRs, especially in the case of drugs known to affect specific organ systems (e.g., liver function tests for hepatotoxicity).
d. **Electronic Health Records (EHRs):** Utilizing electronic health record systems to track and analyse patient data for patterns of adverse effects, integration of decision support tools in EHRs to assist in identifying potential ADRs.
e. **Pharmacovigilance Programs:** Involvement in national or regional pharmacovigilance programs that collect, analyze, and disseminate information on ADRs; collaboration with regulatory agencies and pharmaceutical companies to share information on emerging safety concerns.

Reporting of Adverse Drug Reactions:
a. **Healthcare Professionals:** Physicians, nurses, pharmacists, and other healthcare providers are responsible for reporting ADRs to relevant authorities by filling out and submitting ADR reporting forms provided by regulatory agencies.
b. **Patients:** Encouraging patients to report ADRs directly to healthcare providers or through consumer reporting systems, some countries have established mechanisms for patients to report ADRs directly to regulatory agencies.
c. **Pharmaceutical Companies:** Manufacturers of pharmaceuticals play a role in monitoring and reporting ADRs identified during clinical trials or post-marketing surveillance, collaborating with regulatory agencies to provide timely and accurate information on ADRs associated with their products.

d. **Regulatory Agencies:** National regulatory agencies, such as the FDA in the United States or the EMA in Europe, have established systems for ADR reporting; a centralized database is often maintained to collect and analyze reports, contributing to ongoing safety assessments.

e. **International Collaboration:** Participation in international pharmacovigilance collaborations, such as the World Health Organization's Global Individual Case Safety Reports (ICSRs) database, facilitates the sharing of ADR information globally.

f. **Incentives for Reporting:** Implementing incentives for healthcare professionals and others involved in the reporting process, such as recognition, continuing education credits, or other rewards.

2.3. Methods in Causality Assessment:

Causality assessment in the context of adverse drug reactions (ADRs) involves determining the likelihood and strength of the relationship between a drug and an observed adverse event. Various methods are employed to assess causality, and these methods help healthcare professionals and regulatory agencies make informed decisions about the safety of a drug.

Some commonly used methods in causality assessment are:

1. The Naranjo Algorithm, which Naranjo et al. developed, offers a structured method for determining the likelihood that a drug and an adverse event are causally related. It assigns scores based on factors such as the temporal relationship, previous patient experience with the drug, dechallenge and rechallenge information, and alternative explanations.

2. World Health Organization (WHO) Causality Categories: The WHO has established standardized causality assessment categories, including certain, probable, possible, unlikely, conditional/unclassified, and unassessable/unclassifiable. These categories help standardize the evaluation process across different settings.

3. Liverpool Causality Assessment Tool (LCAT): LCAT is a causality assessment tool that considers factors such as the temporal relationship, dechallenge and rechallenge information, and the presence of similar reactions with the same drug or class of drugs. It provides a structured framework for healthcare professionals to assign causality categories.

4. Roussel Uclaf Causality Assessment Method (RUCAM): Developed for assessing causality in drug-induced liver injury, RUCAM provides a systematic approach based on different criteria, assigning scores to various elements like temporal relationships, challenge and rechallenge data, risk factors, and alternative causes.

5. Adverse Event Reaction Probability Scale (Baldness Scale): The Baldness Scale is a probabilistic approach to assess causality in drug-induced hepatotoxicity. It considers factors such as temporal relationships, the exclusion of alternative causes, and challenge data.

6. Karch and Lasagna Modification of the Naranjo Scale: An adapted version of the Naranjo Algorithm, this modification incorporates additional criteria and emphasizes the importance of exclusion of alternative causes in causality assessment.

7. Algorithm-Based Approaches: Some algorithms have been developed for specific types of adverse events, such as the algorithm for drug causality in acute pancreatitis (CADIAP), which helps assess the likelihood of drugs causing acute pancreatitis.

8. Bayesian Methods: Bayesian analysis involves statistical methods to estimate the probability of causality by combining prior probabilities with new evidence. These methods can be applied in a variety of contexts, including pharmacovigilance.

Causality assessment often involves a combination of methods and clinical judgment, healthcare professionals and regulatory agencies consider the specific circumstances of each case, including patient history, clinical presentation, temporal relationship, and the presence of alternative explanations, to make informed decisions about the likelihood of a drug causing an adverse event, it's important to note that no single method is universally accepted or applicable to all situations.

2.4. Severity and seriousness assessment:

Assessing the severity and seriousness of adverse drug reactions (ADRs) is critical for ensuring appropriate management and communication of risks associated with the use of medications. These assessments help healthcare professionals, regulatory agencies, and pharmaceutical companies categorize and prioritize ADRs. Here are the key aspects of severity and seriousness assessment:

Severity Assessment includes:

Mild: Symptoms are bothersome but generally do not interfere significantly with daily activities, no or minimal medical intervention is required.

Moderate: Symptoms may require medical attention and can impact daily activities; medical intervention may be necessary to alleviate or manage symptoms.

Severe: Symptoms are intense, significantly affecting the patient's well-being; medical intervention is often required urgently; and the adverse event may be life-threatening.

Life-Threatening: Adverse events that pose an immediate risk to the patient's life require prompt medical intervention to prevent a fatal outcome.

Disabling or Permanent Damage: Adverse events leading to long-term impairment or permanent damage to a specific organ or function can significantly impact the patient's quality of life.

Seriousness Assessment includes:

a. **Serious Adverse Drug Reaction:** Whichever adverse event that results to death or life-threatening, it requires hospitalization and existing of it causes prolongation of hospitalization, results in continual or notable disability or incapacity, or is a physical abnormality or birth defect.

b. **Non-Serious ADR:** Adverse events that do not meet the criteria for seriousness as defined by regulatory authorities may include mild or moderate adverse events that do not result in severe consequences.

Considerations in Severity and Seriousness Assessment includes:
1. **Temporal Relationship:** The timing of the adverse event in relation to drug administration is crucial. Acute and immediate events may be considered more severe.
2. **Reversibility:** assessing whether the adverse event is reversible or if it leads to permanent damage or disability.
3. **Impact on Daily Activities:** Evaluating how the adverse event affects the patient's ability to perform daily tasks and maintain a normal life.
4. **Patient Perspective:** Considering the patient's perspective on the impact of the adverse event and their quality of life.
5. **Clinical Judgment:** Healthcare professionals use their clinical judgment, considering the overall clinical context, to determine the severity and seriousness of an adverse event.
6. **Regulatory Definitions:** Regulatory agencies, such as the U.S. Food and Drug Administration (FDA) or the European Medicines Agency (EMA), provide specific definitions for serious and non-serious adverse events to guide reporting requirements, accurate and standardized severity and seriousness assessments contribute to the overall understanding of a drug's safety profile. They guide healthcare professionals in prioritizing interventions and regulatory agencies in making decisions regarding drug labeling, safety communications, and potential regulatory actions. Regular communication and reporting of such assessments are crucial for maintaining and updating the risk-benefit profile of medications throughout their lifecycle.

Factor	Questions	Score
Drug	*Knowledge about the drug and its possible role*	
	1. Hypothesis, still debated.	+1
	2. A matter of worry, diffused by publication or work in progress.	+2
	3. Causality established.	+3
	Communication about this knowledge	
	1. Reassuring about a lack of danger.	0
	2. Relatively worrying.	+2
	3. Serious cause for concern about presence of danger.	+3
Patient	*Clinical case: Risk factors*	
	1. No risk factor.	0
	2. Hardly detectable risk factor.	+2
	3. Risk factor present and easy to detect.	+3
	Drug management	
	1. Respect of recommendations or lack of precautions has played. Any role in the present case:	0
	2. Recommendation not applicable easily in the present case.	+2
	3. Recommendation easy to apply by the prescriber or the patient, but neglected.	+3
Prescription	*Conditions of prescription*	
	1. Prescription indispensable to the patient.	−12
	2. Questionable, but acceptable prescription.	−4
	3. Inappropriate prescription (needless or completely contraindicated).	+3
	Management of adverse reaction	
	1. Excellent, with prevention of aggravation of the adverse reactions.	0
	2. Inadequate.	+2
	3. Absent, with aggravation of the reactions.	+3

Fig.1: Severity and Seriousness Assessment (Risk Benefit Ratio)

2.5. Predictability and preventability assessment:

Predictability and preventability assessments in the context of adverse drug reactions (ADRs) involve evaluating the likelihood of an ADR occurring and determining the potential for preventing or minimizing its occurrence. These assessments contribute to enhancing patient safety and guiding healthcare professionals in optimizing medication use.

a. Predictability assessment includes:

1. Type A (Augmented) Reactions (i.e., Predictable): These reactions are dose-dependent and directly related to the known pharmacological actions of the drug. Their occurrence can often be anticipated based on the drug's mechanism of action.

2. Type B (Bizarre) Reactions (i.e., Unpredictable): These reactions are not related to the known pharmacological actions of the drug and often involve idiosyncratic responses. They are less predictable and subject to individual genetic influences.

3. Patient-Related Factors: Consideration of patient-specific factors such as age, gender, genetics, and pre-existing medical conditions that may influence the predictability of ADRs.

4. Drug-Related Factors: Examination of drug characteristics, including pharmacokinetics, pharmacodynamics, and the potential for drug interactions, to assess the predictability of ADRs.

5. Pre-existing Knowledge: The availability of prior information on similar ADRs associated with the drug or class of drugs can enhance predictability.

b. Preventability Assessment:

1. Avoidability of Exposure: Evaluation of whether the ADR could have been avoided by modifying the dose, route of administration, or duration of drug therapy.

2. Patient Education: Assessing the role of patient education in preventing ADRs by informing patients about potential side effects, the importance of adherence to medication regimens, and how to recognize and report adverse events.

3. Monitoring Strategies: Implementation of monitoring strategies, including laboratory tests or clinical assessments, to identify early signs of potential ADRs and enable timely intervention.

4. Risk Mitigation Strategies: Utilization of risk mitigation strategies, such as dose adjustments in vulnerable populations or the use of alternative medications with a lower risk of specific ADRs.

5. Healthcare Professional Training: ensuring that healthcare professionals are adequately trained to recognize and manage ADRs, as well as to educate patients on the potential risks associated with medications.

6. Decision Support Systems: Integration of clinical decision support systems to provide healthcare professionals with real-time information on potential drug interactions, contraindications, and dose adjustments.

7. Pharmacovigilance Programs: Participation in pharmacovigilance programs to systematically collect, assess, and disseminate information on ADRs facilitates proactive measures to prevent similar events.

8. Regulatory Actions: Regulatory agencies may take preventive actions, such as updating drug labels, issuing warnings, or implementing risk management plans, based on the available evidence of preventable ADRs, both predictability and preventability assessments contribute to optimizing the risk-benefit profile of medications, these assessments inform healthcare decision-making, guide regulatory actions, and enhance patient safety.

2.6. Management of adverse drug reactions:

The management of adverse drug reactions (ADRs) involves a comprehensive approach to address the symptoms, prevent further harm, and improve patient outcomes. The specific management strategies depend on the nature and severity of the ADR. Here are general principles and approaches for managing adverse drug reactions:

a. Discontinuation of the causative drug: The primary and immediate step in managing an ADR is to discontinue the suspected causative drug. This helps prevent further exposure and reduces the risk of exacerbating the adverse event.

b. Supportive care: Provide supportive care to manage symptoms and maintain the patient's overall well-being. This may include hydration, pain management, antiemetics, or other supportive measures, depending on the nature of the adverse event.

c. Specific antidotes or reversal agents: In some cases, specific antidotes or reversal agents may be available to counteract the effects of the causative drug. For example, naloxone can be used as an antidote for opioid overdose.

d. Symptomatic treatment: Address specific symptoms associated with the ADR through symptomatic treatment. For instance, antihistamines for allergic reactions, bronchodilators for respiratory symptoms, or topical treatments for skin reactions.

e. Dechallenge and rechallenge: If appropriate and under close medical supervision, dechallenge (stopping the drug) and rechallenge (restarting the drug) may be considered to confirm the causative role of the drug in the ADR. However, this approach is not suitable for all situations and should be done cautiously.

f. Management of allergic reactions: Allergic reactions may require immediate intervention with antihistamines, corticosteroids, and, in severe cases, epinephrine (adrenaline). Anaphylaxis is a medical emergency and requires prompt administration of epinephrine.

g. Consultation with specialists: In complex cases or when the ADR affects specific organ systems, consulting with specialists such as allergists, dermatologists, or hepatologists may be necessary for expert management.

h. Monitoring and follow-up: Regular monitoring and follow-up are essential to assess the progress of ADR management and to detect any new or worsening symptoms. Adjustments to the treatment plan may be necessary based on ongoing assessments.

i. Documentation and reporting: Thoroughly document the ADR, including details of the patient's medical history, symptoms, and the management plan. Report the ADR to relevant regulatory authorities as part of pharmacovigilance efforts.

j. Patient education: Educate the patient about the ADR, the importance of medication adherence, and the signs and symptoms that warrant immediate medical attention. This empowers patients to actively participate in their healthcare.

k. Prevention of recurrence: Identify and implement preventive measures to avoid the recurrence of similar ADRs in the future. This may involve choosing alternative medications, adjusting doses, or employing additional monitoring strategies.

l. Collaboration with regulatory authorities: Healthcare professionals and organizations should collaborate with regulatory authorities to contribute to the ongoing assessment of drug safety profiles and update product labeling as needed.

ADR Monitoring Form

M ☐ F ☐ Name of the Patient .... HN ....

Date of ADR occurring ....

Adverse events ....

....

Suspected drug(s) ....

....

Suspected drug group ....

Organ affected ....

Causality assessment:

☐ Highly   ☐ Probable   ☐ Possible   ☐ Unlikely

Type of ADR:

☐ Type A   ☐ Type B

Mechanism of an ADR:

☐ Side effect   ☐ Toxicity   ☐ Secondary effect   ☐ Drug interaction

☐ Intolerance   ☐ Allergy   ☐ Pseudo-allergy   ☐ Idiosyncracy

Severity of an ADR:

☐ Level 1: An ADR occurred but required no change in treatment with the suspected drug.

☐ Level 2: The ADR required that treatment with the suspected drug be continued, discontinued, or changed. No antidote or other treatment required. No increase in LOS.

☐ Level 3: The ADR required that treatment with suspected drug be continued, discontinued, or changed, and/or an antidote or other treatment was required. No increase in LOS.

☐ Level 4: Any level 3 ADR which increases LOS by at least one day.

☐ Level 5: Any level 4 ADR which required intensive medical care.

☐ Level 6: The ADR caused permanent harm to the patient.

☐ Level 7: The ADR either directly or indirectly led to the death of the patient.

Preventability assessment

1. Was the drug involved in the ADR not considered appropriate for the patient's clinical condition?
2. Was the dose, route, and frequency of administration not appropriate for the patient's age, weight and disease state?
3. Was required therapeutic drug monitoring or other necessary laboratory test not performed?
4. Was there a history of allergy or previous reaction to the drug?
5. Was a drug interaction involved in the reaction?
6. Was a toxic serum drug level documented?
7. Was poor compliance involved in the reaction?

☐ Yes, if one or more of above are chosen   ☐ No

Fig. 2: ADR Monitoring form

Chapter 3
Basic terminologies used in pharmacovigilance

It is essential to tailor the Basic terminologies used in pharmacovigilance:

1. Pharmacovigilance: Such activities related for the detection, assessment, understanding, and prevention of any other drug-related problems or adverse effects. understanding these terms is essential for professionals working in drug safety, regulatory affairs, and healthcare.

2. Adverse Drug Reaction (ADR): A verbal or written answer to a medicine that is unintended and potentially harmful, occurring at doses normally used for the treatment, prevention, or diagnosis of a disease.

3. Suspected Adverse Drug Reaction (SADR): Any adverse event suspected to be related to the use of a medicine.

4. Serious Adverse Event (SAE) or Serious Adverse Drug Reaction (SADR): Any adverse event that results in death or life-threatening it requires inpatient hospitalization or prolongation of existing hospitalization, that results in significant or persistent disability, or is a congenital anomaly or birth defect.

5. Signal: A SADR that is suspected ADR to be caused by a medicine and is identified during the pharmacovigilance activities; information that suggests potentially causal association or a new aspect association between an intervention or an event.

6. Post-marketing surveillance: The monitoring of the safety of a drug after it has been approved and is available on the market.

7. Causality: The relationship between an adverse event and the suspected medicinal product leads to the conclusion that the drug caused the adverse event.

8. Benefit-risk assessment: The process of evaluating the expected benefit of a medicine against its potential risks.

9. Risk management plan: A comprehensive plan to identify, evaluate, and reduce the risks associated with a medicinal product throughout its lifecycle

10. Risk Minimization Action Plan (RiskMAP): A plan to identify, evaluate, and reduce the risks associated with a medicinal product.

11. Pharmacovigilance System Master File (PSMF): A document that provides a comprehensive overview of the pharmacovigilance system of a medicinal product.

12. Risk Evaluation and Mitigation Strategies (REMS): A strategy to identify, evaluate, and reduce the risks associated with a medicinal product.

13. Aggregate report: A report that summarizes the safety data of a medicinal product on an aggregate level.

14. Good Pharmacovigilance Practice (GVP): A set of measures and processes to ensure the systematic monitoring of medicinal products and the detection, assessment, understanding and prevention of adverse drug-related problems.

15. Patient safety: The prevention of harm to patients during the provision of healthcare, including the use of medicinal products.

16. MedDRA (Medical Dictionary for Drug Regulatory Activities): A medical standardized terminology developed by the International Council for Harmonization of Technical Requirements for Pharmaceuticals for Human Use (ICH) for the classification of adverse term events.

17. Individual Case Safety Report (ICSR): A report that includes information on a single case of an adverse drug reaction, usually submitted by healthcare professionals, patients, or pharmaceutical companies.

18. Regulatory Reporting: The obligation to report adverse drug reactions to regulatory authorities according to established timelines and criteria.

19. Periodic Safety Update Report (PSUR) or Periodic Benefit-Risk Evaluation Report (PBRER): A regulatory document submitted at defined intervals that provides a comprehensive analysis of the benefit-risk profile of a medicinal product.

20. Regulatory Authority: A government agency responsible for the regulation, approval, and oversight of medicinal products within a specific jurisdiction.

21. Risk Minimization Measures: Strategies implemented to minimize the occurrence or impact of identified risks associated with a medicinal product.

22. Common Terminology Criteria for Adverse Events (CTCAE) and Center for Drug Evaluation and Research (CDER).

3.1. Terminologies of adverse medication-related events:

Terminologies related to adverse medication-related events encompass a range of terms used to describe various aspects of incidents, errors, and negative outcomes associated with the use of medications.

a. Adverse Drug Event (ADE): Any injury resulting from the use of a drug, including medication errors, adverse drug reactions, overdoses, and allergic reactions.

b. Medication Error: Any event that may preventable can cause or lead to inappropriate medication use or harm of patient, while the control of medication is in of the healthcare professional, patient, or consumer.

c. Near Miss: An event that did not cause harm but had the potential to do so. It is a close call that could have resulted in an adverse medication event but was intercepted before reaching the patient.

d. Prescribing Error: An error in the prescription of a medication, such as incorrect dosage, route, frequency, or drug selection.

e. Dispensing Error: Mistakes that occur during the preparation and distribution of a medication, often involving errors in labeling, packaging, or dispensing the wrong drug.

f. Administration Error: Mistakes made during the process of administering a medication, including errors in dose, route, timing, or the patient to whom the medication is given.

g. Monitoring Error: Failure to appropriately monitor a patient's response to medication, leading to a failure to detect and address adverse effects or therapeutic failure.

h. Adherence Issues: non-compliance or non-adherence to prescribed medication regimens by patients, which can lead to suboptimal treatment outcomes.

i. Polypharmacy: The use of multiple medications by a patient, which may increase the risk of adverse drug interactions, side effects, and medication-related issues.

j. Drug-Drug Interaction: Effects that occur when two or more drugs interact with each other, potentially leading to altered therapeutic effects, increased toxicity, or reduced efficacy of one or both drugs.

k. Overdose: The administration of a medication at a dosage higher than recommended, leading to harmful effects that can be acute or chronic.

l. Under-dose: Administering a medication at a lower dosage than recommended, potentially resulting in treatment failure or an inadequate therapeutic effect.

m. Tolerance: A reduced response to a drug over time, requiring an increase in dosage to achieve the same therapeutic effect.

n. Withdrawal: The onset of symptoms when a medication is discontinued, often occurring due to physical or psychological dependence.

o. Black Box Warning: A warning on the labeling of a medication to alert healthcare providers and patients about serious or life-threatening risks associated with the drug.

p. Risk Evaluation and Mitigation Strategy (REMS): A strategy implemented by the U.S. Food and Drug Administration (FDA) to manage known or potential serious risks associated with a medication.

3.2. Regulatory terminologies

Regulatory terminologies are specific terms and phrases used in the context of regulatory affairs, which involve the processes and activities related to the development, approval, and post-marketing oversight of pharmaceuticals, medical devices, and other health-related products.

1. Regulatory Authority: A government agency or body responsible for regulating and overseeing the approval, marketing, and safety of drugs, medical devices, and other healthcare products within a specific jurisdiction, an official regulatory authority's approval for the marketing and sale of a drug or medical device is known as a marketing authorization (or approval).

2. A new drug application (NDA) is a formal application submitted to a regulatory authority seeking approval for the marketing and sale of a new drug.

3. Biologics License Application (BLA): An application submitted to a regulatory authority for the approval of a biological product, including vaccines, blood components, and gene therapies.

4. Abbreviated New Drug Application (ANDA): An application submitted to a regulatory authority for the approval of a generic version of a previously approved drug.

5. Investigational New Drug (IND): A regulatory submission to a regulatory authority seeking permission to conduct clinical trials with an investigational drug.

6. Clinical Trial Application (CTA): A submission to a regulatory authority seeking approval to conduct clinical trials with a new drug or medical device.

7. Good Clinical Practice (GCP): A set of international ethical and scientific quality standards for the design, conduct, performance, recording, monitoring, auditing, analysis and reporting of clinical trials.

8. Good Laboratory Practice (GLP): A set of principles and practices ensuring the quality and integrity of non-clinical laboratory studies supporting research and development activities.

9. Good Manufacturing Practice (GMP): a system ensuring that products are consistently produced and controlled according to quality standards throughout the manufacturing process.

10. Post-Marketing Surveillance (PMS): the monitoring of the safety and effectiveness of a drug or medical device after it has been approved and is available on the market.

11. Pharmacovigilance: the activities related to the detection, assessment, understanding, and prevention of adverse effects or drug-related problems.

12. Quality Management System (QMS): a set of policies, processes, and procedures required for planning and execution in the core business area of an organization.

13. Regulatory Affairs (RA): The department within a pharmaceutical or medical device company responsible for ensuring compliance with regulatory requirements and facilitating the approval and marketing of products.

14. Risk Management Plan (RMP): A comprehensive plan to identify, characterize, and minimize risks associated with a medicinal product throughout its lifecycle.

15. Fast Track, Breakthrough Therapy, and Orphan Drug Designation: Special designations granted by regulatory authorities to expedite the development and approval of drugs targeting serious or rare diseases.

16. Periodic Safety Update Report (PSUR) or Periodic Benefit-Risk Evaluation Report (PBRER): a regulatory document submitted at defined intervals that provides a comprehensive analysis of the benefit-risk profile of a medicinal product.

Unit 2

Chapter 4
Classification of drugs and diseases

Drugs can be described in a number of ways, but the most common ones represent grouping them according to their pharmacological effect, chemical makeup, mode of action, or therapeutic application.

1. **Pharmacological Effect:** Medication can be categorized based on how it affects the body. For instance, antibiotics (fight bacterial infections), analgesics (relieve pain), antihypertensives (reduce blood pressure), etc.

2. **Chemical Structure:** Based on their chemical makeup, drugs can be divided into several categories. For example, steroids, benzodiazepines, and opioids.

3. **Mechanism of Action:** This category considers how medications function within the body. While some medications, like beta-blockers, work by attaching to particular receptors, others work by inhibiting enzymes or affecting particular processes.

When it comes to classifying diseases, this usually entails putting them in groups according to a variety of factors:

1. Diseases can be categorized according to their etiology, or cause, which includes infectious diseases brought on by pathogens, hereditary diseases, autoimmune diseases, etc.

2. Anatomical Site: Some classifications, such as those for neurological conditions, respiratory diseases, cardiac conditions, etc., are based on the organ or system that has been affected.

3. Pathophysiology: This describes the altered functions linked to an illness. Diseases could be grouped, for instance, according to the underlying biological mechanisms—such as

inflammation or hormone imbalances—that give rise to the condition.

4. Severity and Duration: Another way to categorize a condition is based on how severe it is (acute or chronic) or how long it lasts (short-term or long-term).

4.1. Drug categorization based on anatomy, therapeutics, and chemistry:
The Anatomical Therapeutic Chemical (ATC) method classifies pharmaceuticals according to their chemical makeup, anatomical site of action, and therapeutic usage.

1. Anatomical Classification: According to the organ or system that a drug primarily affects, medicines are categorized into several groups by the ATC. Here are a few instances:

A. Alimentary Tract and Metabolism: Medications pertaining to the metabolism and digestive tract.

B. Blood and Blood-Forming Organs: Drugs that impact the blood or blood constituents.

C. Cardiovascular System: Medications for disorders of the heart and blood vessels.

D. Dermatological: drugs for conditions relating to the skin.

G. Genito-Urinary System and Sex Hormones: Substances pertaining to the urinary and reproductive systems.

N. Nervous System: pharmaceuticals for ailments of the nervous system.

R stands for respiratory system; medications for respiratory ailments.

S. Sensory Organs: Medications for problems with the eyes, ears, and other sensory organs. 2.

2. Therapeutic Classification: This system of classification divides medications into groups according to their primary indication or therapeutic usage. As an illustration, anti-infectives are prescriptions meant to treat illnesses brought on by fungi, viruses, bacteria, etc. Analgesics are painkilling drugs. Antidepressants are medications that treat depression. Antihypertensives are blood pressure-lowering drugs. Antineoplastics: anticancer medications.

3. Classification of Chemicals: This classification is predicated on the chemical makeup or structure of pharmaceuticals. It comprises several groups, including beta-lactam antibiotics, which consist of cephalosporins and penicillins. NSAIDs, or nonsteroidal anti-inflammatory drugs, include aspirin and ibuprofen. ACE Inhibitors: Drugs used to treat hypertension that block the angiotensin-converting enzyme. Statins are medications used to reduce cholesterol. Benzodiazepines: sedatives and anxiolytics, such as lorazepam and diazepam.

4.2. The International Classification of Diseases: It is a widely utilized framework for classifying illnesses, medical ailments, and associated problems. The World Health Organization (WHO) is in charge of maintaining and publishing it. The ICD's main objectives are:

1. Clinical Use: To categorize illnesses and other health issues noted on a variety of vital and health records, including hospital and death certificate records.

2. Research and epidemiology: To examine global health trends and data to help determine the frequency, distribution, and incidence of illnesses and ailments.

3. Health management and resource allocation: To support the planning of healthcare services and the distribution of resources according to the prevalence of diseases in various geographic areas.

The most recent revision of the ICD, as of the most recent update in January 2022, is the ICD-10. The alphanumeric classification system is divided into chapters, each of which focuses on a particular body system or group of diseases. The ICD is updated and revised on a regular basis to reflect changes in disease patterns and advances in medical science. For example:

Chapter I: Several parasitic and viral illnesses, Chapter II: Cancers and Neoplasms, Chapter III: Disorders of the Blood and Organs that Form Blood Endocrine, nutritional, and metabolic disorders (Chapter

IV), Chapter V: Disorders of the mind, behaviour, and neurodevelopment, Chapter VI: Nervous system disorders, Chapter VII: Ocular and adnexal diseases, Chapter VIII: Ear and mastoid process disorders, Chapter IX: Circulatory system disorders, Chapter X: Respiratory system diseases, Chapter XI: Digestive System Disorders, Chapter XII: Skin Conditions, Chapter XIII: Conditions affecting the connective tissue and musculoskeletal system, Chapter XIV: Genitourinary System Disorders, Chapter XV: The puerperium, delivery, and pregnancy, Chapter XVI: A few ailments that have their roots in the perinatal stage Congenital deformities, malformations, and chromosomal anomalies are covered in Chapter XVII, Chapter XVIII: Unusual clinical and laboratory results, symptoms, and indications that are not otherwise categorized, Chapter XIX: Contamination, harm, and additional repercussions from outside sources, Chapter XX: External Factors Contributing to Morbidity and Death, Chapter XXI: Variables affecting health status and utilization of medical services.

4.3. Daily defined doses (DDDs):
This is the standardized measurement tool used in pharmacology and pharmaceutical research to compare the consumption of various medications or active substances. The World Health Organization (WHO) developed the concept of DDDs to analyze drug utilization and medication consumption patterns globally; however, it should not be interpreted as a patient's recommended or prescribed daily dose. Instead, it is a standardized measurement tool to help compare the consumption of various drugs or drug classes. Each DDD is defined for a specific active substance, and it is frequently based on the average maintenance dose used for the main indication in adults. For the majority of medications, it is usually stated in terms of grams or milligrams per day, though depending on the drug, it may also be specified in other units. For instance, the DDD for a specific antibiotic may be one gram per day, while the DDD for an antihypertensive medication may be fifty milligrams per day.

DDDs serve the following purposes:

1. Comparative studies: To assess how various medications are used in different areas, countries, or within a therapeutic class.

2. Pharmacoepidemiology: To examine differences in prescribing procedures and track drug consumption patterns.

3. Health policy and resource allocation: By comprehending drug usage trends, policies and resources for healthcare can be made more effective.

4.4. Worldwide "Internationally Non-proprietary Names" (INN) for pharmaceutical substances or active ingredients in drugs:

The INNs are standardized, internationally recognized names for pharmacological substances. The idea behind INN is to give everyone, everywhere, in whatever language or location, a common, distinctive, and instantly identifiable name. The World Health Organization (WHO) created these names. INNs are especially helpful in the following ways:

1. Standardization: INNs give each active pharmaceutical ingredient a single, distinct name, minimizing confusion that could result from using different brand names in different nations.

2. Medical Communication: They serve as a global communication hub for researchers, pharmacists, healthcare providers, and regulatory bodies.

3. Regulatory and Scientific Use: For coherence and clarity, INNs are employed in pharmacopoeias, scientific publications, and drug registration. INNs are chosen in accordance with strict guidelines and taken into consideration for a variety of reasons. Clarity and ease of pronouncing in various languages, lack of uncertainty or potential confusion with other names, and international acceptability and recognition are a few examples. For example, acetaminophen, also known as paracetamol, is the common name for a medication that is widely used to reduce fever and relieve pain. While INNs give a defined designation for the active component, different pharmaceutical companies may market medications with the same active ingredient under different brand names. Another example is Ibuprofen, which is the common name while its INN remains "ibuprofen." This promotes manufacturer competition while maintaining uniformity in identifying the drug's active ingredient.

Chapter 5
Codes and drug dictionaries in pharmacovigilance

Drug dictionaries and coding systems are essential for standardizing and organizing data regarding medications and adverse events in pharmacovigilance, the monitoring and evaluation of pharmaceutical products' safety.

1. The World Health Organization maintains the ***WHO Drug Dictionary (WHO-DD),*** which includes information on medications such as brand names, active ingredients, codes for specific drugs, and International Non-proprietary Names (INNs). Pharmacovigilance uses it extensively to standardize drug information.

2. Information on adverse events is encoded using standardized medical terminology called **MedDRA (Medical Dictionary for Drug Regulatory Activities).** With its vocabulary of illnesses, symptoms, and adverse responses, MedDRA makes it possible to report and analyze adverse events consistently across databases and geographical areas.

Coding Frameworks:

a. **The Anatomical Therapeutic Chemical Classification System**, or ATC classification system, groups medications according to their chemical makeup and intended medicinal function. In pharmacovigilance, it is employed for uniform drug identification and classification.

b. **The WHO Adverse Reaction Terminology**, or WHO-ART, is a coding system that is used to encode adverse responses and offers standardized terminology for reporting and examining side effects related to drugs.

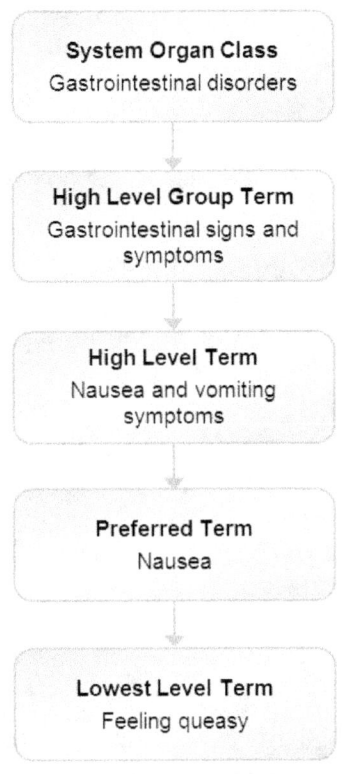

Fig. 3. MedDRA Hierarchy

Pharmacovigilance role:
a. Data standardization: Coding schemes and drug dictionaries aid in the organization and standardization of data about prescription drugs and side effects. This standardization makes it possible to conduct consistent reporting and analysis across various databases and geographical areas.
b. Signal Detection: Pharmacovigilance professionals can spot possible safety signals or trends connected to certain medications or drug classes by classifying data using standardized nomenclature and coding.
c. Regulatory Reporting: These systems help with regulatory judgments about drug safety by making it easier to report adverse occurrences to regulatory agencies using standardized nomenclature.
d. Data Analysis and Research: To help guarantee patient safety, standardized drug dictionaries and coding systems facilitate efficient

data analysis, research, and comparison of safety profiles among various medications.

5.1. Terminologies for adverse reactions defined by the World Health Organization (WHO): The WHO has created a number of categories and terminologies that are particularly focused on adverse responses linked to medication. The following is some unnamed WHO adverse reaction terminology that helps standardize the reporting, documenting, and analysis of drug-related adverse events:

1. The WHO Adverse Reaction Terminology, or WHO-ART, is a standardized terminology dictionary that is used to code adverse drug-related events. It offers a common language for characterizing and disclosing negative responses. The terminologies used by WHO-ART encompass a broad spectrum of adverse events, such as drug-related symptoms, signs, illnesses, and clinical outcomes.

2. Medical Dictionary for Regulatory Activities (MedDRA), MedDRA is an extensive medical terminology created with input from the WHO by the International Conference on Harmonization (ICH). A wide range of standardized words and codes describing adverse events, such as symptoms, illnesses, and clinical findings connected to medical items, including medications, are included in MedDRA.

3. The WHO Drug Dictionary contains information on side effects and reactions related to certain pharmaceuticals, even though its main concentration is on drug nomenclature and identification. This dictionary supports pharmacovigilance efforts by making it easier to identify and categorize drugs and the side effects that go along with them in a consistent manner.

Standardization is a key component of pharmacovigilance, as these terminologies offer standardized vocabularies that facilitate uniform reporting and analysis of adverse events across various databases, geographical areas, and healthcare systems.

a. Safety Monitoring: They make it possible to efficiently track and analyze data on drug safety, which helps to identify possible side effects linked to prescription drugs.

b. Regulatory Reporting: By facilitating the reporting of adverse events to regulatory bodies, standardized terminology aids in the evaluation of medication safety profiles.

c. Research and Analysis: By giving researchers a consistent language to describe adverse events, these terminologies facilitate the comparison and analysis of safety data from various studies and populations.

5.2. MedDRA (Medical Dictionary for Regulatory Activities) and Standardized MedDRA queries:

MedDRA is a standardized medical terminology used for be responsible for producing and categorizing adverse event data related to medical products, mostly in pharmaceuticals. It is extensively employed in regulatory and pharmacovigilance functions, standardized MedDRA Queries (SMQs) are word subsets taken from the larger MedDRA lexicon that are designed to make it easier to find and retrieve particular sets of adverse events.

1. MedDRA:

Goal: MedDRA provides a standardized language for the description and group of clinical findings, illnesses, signs and symptoms, even the adverse events related to medical items (drugs, vaccines, devices, etc.). Structure: The phrases are grouped from general to specialized in a hierarchy that makes it possible to code and classify unfavorable events in great detail. Coding Procedure: To enable uniform and standardized reporting across various databases and healthcare systems, adverse events that are reported are coded using MedDRA terminology.

2. MedDRA Standardized Queries (SMQs):

Goal: SMQs are pre-arranged collections of MedDRA terms that concentrate on particular ailments, signs, or occurrences. These queries are designed to make it easier to obtain and analyze adverse event data for particular uses. A large number of SMQs cover hepatic injury, cardiac failure, renal injury, psychiatric disorders, and other medical illnesses and events. Specific MedDRA terminology pertaining to the ailment or incident is included in each SMQ. Use: By enabling users to search databases using these predetermined groupings, SMQs facilitate the systematic study of adverse event data by facilitating the quick and easy identification and retrieval of pertinent information.

Pharmacovigilance's importance:
a. Data Analysis: Pharmacovigilance specialists can quickly identify and assess particular groups of medication-related adverse events with the help of SMQs, which aid in targeted analysis.
b. Signal Detection: They assist in the identification of patterns or safety signals connected to specific medical problems or drug-related incidents.
c. Regulatory Reporting: To give more thorough and uniform information regarding particular adverse events connected to medications, SMQs might be utilized in regulatory reporting.

5.3. The World Health Organization (WHO) has created and is maintaining the WHO Drug Dictionary:

A comprehensive resource that offers standardized information about pharmacological chemicals and therapeutic products:
1. The goal of standardization is to create a worldwide standard for drug names, coding, and identification. This standardization facilitates uniform drug recording and communication among various healthcare systems and geographical areas.
2. Identification and Classification: Information regarding brand names, active ingredients, strengths, dosage forms, International Non-proprietary Names (INNs), and other relevant information about pharmaceutical goods is included in the dictionary.

Important characteristics:
a. WHO has given generic names for pharmaceutical substances known as International Non-proprietary Names (INNs) in order to guarantee that the names of the active ingredients are known throughout the world. INNs are a crucial component of drug identification, according to the WHO Drug Dictionary.

b. Drug Coding: Each drug entry in the dictionary has a unique code that makes it possible to clearly identify and categorize pharmaceuticals.

c. Therapeutic Classification: It helps classify pharmaceuticals according to their indications or mechanisms of action by providing information on the pharmacological and therapeutic uses of drugs.

d. Dose Forms and Strengths: Details on various dose forms (tablets, capsules, injections, etc.) and pharmaceutical strengths are provided, enabling accurate identification.

Relevance to Healthcare:

a. Medical Communication: Standardized drug information is provided, which enables efficient communication between researchers, pharmacists, healthcare providers, and regulatory agencies.

b. Drug Safety and Pharmacovigilance: By guaranteeing correct drug identification and reporting in adverse event monitoring and drug safety evaluations, it supports pharmacovigilance activities.

c. Regulatory Use: For uniformity and accuracy in medication identification and classification, this information is utilized in regulatory submissions, drug approvals, and global health authorities' monitoring.

d. Research and Clinical Practice: Ensures precision and clarity in drug identification by offering a standardized reference for researchers and clinicians to use when referring to or prescribing drugs.

5.4. The European Medicines Agency (EMA) is in charge of the EudraVigilance Medicinal Product Dictionary (EVMPD): Which is a centralized European database, it is a point of reference for pharmacovigilance activities and regulatory procedures within the European Union (EU) and contains comprehensive information about medicinal products marketed in the European Economic Area (EEA).

a. Goal of Regulatory Compliance: The EU legislation's regulatory criteria for the thorough and uniform recording of medical product information were met by the establishment of the EVMPD.

b. Reporting on Pharmacovigilance: It acts as a central repository for comprehensive information on pharmaceuticals, facilitating the reporting and observation of side effects connected to these drugs.

c. Important Features: Medicinal Product Information: The EVMPD includes a wealth of information regarding pharmaceuticals, such as: pharmaceutical form; active ingredients; strengths and dosage forms; facts about marketing authorization; packaging; and manufacturer information.

d. Standardization: The purpose of the EEA's EVMPD is to harmonize and standardize the recording and interchange of information on medical products. Pharmacovigilance Support: By offering thorough and consistent data, this service makes it easier to identify the medications that are mentioned in adverse event reports.

Pharmacovigilance's importance: 1. Regulatory Compliance: In order to maintain compliance with EU rules, marketing authorization holders located in the European Economic Area (EEA) must provide the EVMPD with accurate and up-to-date information about their pharmaceutical products.

2. Adverse Event Reporting: Facilitates precise drug identification and classification in adverse event reports, supporting efficient safety and pharmacovigilance.

3. Enables regulatory and pharmacovigilance efforts by promoting data consistency and transparency in medical product information throughout the European Economic Area (EEA).

4. Information sharing: encourages regulatory agencies to communicate and work together on drug safety evaluations by supporting the exchange of standardized medical product information.

Chapter 6
Pharmacovigilance information resources

Accessing trustworthy and thorough information sources is essential for pharmacovigilance in order to track and assess the safety of pharmaceuticals.

a. Systems and Databases

b. Eudra-Vigilance is a single database for the gathering and handling of reports of suspected adverse drug reactions throughout the European Economic Area (EEA), and it is supervised by the European Medicines Agency (EMA).

c. FDA Adverse Event Reporting System (FAERS): Reviews adverse events and drug errors filed by reporters, consumers, healthcare providers, and manufacturers are stored in the FDA database in the United States.

d. The World Health Organization's (WHO) global database for gathering and examining reports of suspected adverse drug reactions from all across the world is called VigiBase, and it is run by the Uppsala Monitoring Centre (UMC).

e. National Pharmacovigilance Centers: Numerous nations have national pharmacovigilance centers or databases of their own, which gather and examine adverse event information on a national basis.

Books & Publications for Reference:

A comprehensive reference source offering information on pharmaceuticals and medicines globally, including pharmacological data and therapeutic use, is:

a. Guidelines for Good Pharmacovigilance Practice (GVP): Disseminated by regulatory bodies including the FDA and EMA, these guidelines offer criteria and suggestions for pharmacovigilance operations.

b. Martindale: The Complete Drug Reference.

c. Pharmacovigilance Journals: Research articles, case studies, and updates in pharmacovigilance are published in academic and professional journals such as Drug Safety, Pharmacoepidemiology and Drug Safety, and the Journal of Pharmacovigilance.

Web-Based Resources:

  a. MedWatch: An FDA-provided website that provides safety alerts, revisions to safety labels, and additional safety-related data on medications and therapeutic biologics.

  b. WHO Pharmaceuticals Newsletter: Delivers global updates on pharmacovigilance initiatives, regulatory affairs, and drug safety data.

  c. The European Medicines Agency (EMA): Enable databases, reports, and guidance materials about pharmacovigilance and drug safety in the EU.

  d. The Uppsala Monitoring Centre (UMC) offers reports, training materials, and access to VigiBase, among other pharmacovigilance technologies.

  e. Regulations, Reports, and Recommendations: EMA Pharmacovigilance Risk Assessment Committee (PRAC) Reports and recommendations on pharmaceutical safety and risk assessments.

  f. FDA Drug Safety Alerts and Communications: Notifications to the public about drug-related safety concerns, recalls, and advisories.

Rudimentary drug information sources: There are a number of trustworthy sources that offer crucial information on drugs while looking for basic drug information. Here are a few popular ones:

Online Drug Databases: Drugs.com provides a thorough drug database with details on dosage, interactions, adverse effects, and drug uses. Prescription and over-the-counter drugs are included.

a. MedlinePlus: The National Library of Medicine provides information on medications, including uses, side effects, and descriptions that are easy for patients to understand.

b. RxList provides a database of both prescription and over-the-counter drugs, together with information on their uses, interactions, side effects, and cautions.

Official internet pages: 1. FDA Drug Information: Drug labels, safety alerts, and prescription guidelines are just a few of the resources the U.S. The Food and Drug Administration makes available information regarding authorized medications. 2. EMA Medicines: Public evaluation reports and summaries of product characteristics are available, along with information on medicines allowed inside the European Union, from the European Medicines Agency.

Smartphone Applications: Epocrates: A popular tool among medical professionals, it offers details on drugs, such as dosage, interactions, and recommended uses. Comprehensive drug information, including dosage, adverse effects, interactions, and clinical news, is available on Medscape. Textbooks on pharmacology: Goodman & Gilman's The Pharmacological Basis of Therapeutics: An esteemed resource offering comprehensive details on pharmacology and pharmacological effects. Bertram Katzung's Basic and Clinical Pharmacology provides key information on drugs as well as basic pharmacological ideas.

Additional Sources: Pharmaceutical manufacturers provide prescription information about drugs in the form of package inserts that include details on dose, usage, side effects, and warnings. Pharmacist Consultation: For basic drug information, pharmacists are incredibly knowledgeable and easily available. They can answer particular queries and offer advice on drugs.

Specific tools for controlling, recording, and comprehending adverse drug reactions (ADRs) include pharmacovigilance databases, which are designed to help with these tasks.

1. VigiBase (UMC): The global database for adverse drug reactions maintained by the World Health Organization. It compiles data from numerous national pharmacovigilance hub across the planet.
2. The FDA's database of adverse event reports, prescription errors, and product quality concerns that are filed with the agency is called the FDA Adverse Event Reporting System (FAERS).
3. The European database EudraVigilance is used by the European Medicines Agency (EMA) to gather and examine any adverse reaction reports.

Specialist Publications and Journals: a. Medication Safety: Research articles, reviews, and case studies are published in this peer-reviewed magazine that covers all facets of medication safety and pharmacovigilance. b. The journal Therapeutic Innovation & Regulatory Science (TIRS) publishes reviews and research articles on subjects related to drug safety and regulatory science innovation in therapeutics.

Reports and Guidelines for Pharmacovigilance: a. ICH Guidelines: The standard "International Council for Harmonization of Technical Requirements for Pharmaceuticals for Human Use" (ICH) make available guidelines that govern pharmacovigilance methodologies and methods.

b. PRAC Recommendations (EMA): documents and suggestions pertaining to safety concerns and drug risk assessments that are issued by the EMA's Pharmacovigilance Risk Assessment Committee (PRAC).

Resources for Online Pharmacovigilance: The Uppsala Monitoring Centre (UMC) provides information on pharmacovigilance and adverse medication reactions, including articles, tools, and resources. WHO Pharmaceuticals Newsletter: Delivers global updates on pharmacovigilance initiatives, regulatory affairs, and drug safety data.

Portals for Reporting Adverse Events: a. The FDA's MedWatch program enables consumers and medical professionals to report severe issues, including adverse reactions, with medical products. b. The Yellow Card Scheme (MHRA) enables individuals in the UK to report potential adverse drug reactions or side effects,

Targeted Instruction and Training: ***Workshops and Courses on Pharmacovigilance:*** A number of establishments and associations provide specific training sessions and seminars on ADR tracking, signal identification, and pharmacovigilance procedures. Pharmacovigilance Forums and Networks: Attending conferences, forums, and professional networks devoted to pharmacovigilance facilitates the sharing of information and experiences on adverse drug reactions. Creating a pharmacovigilance program entails putting in place the procedures and mechanisms needed to track, evaluate, and oversee the safety of pharmaceuticals over the course of their whole lives.

Chapter 7

Establishing pharmacovigilance program

Consider the following actions when starting a pharmacovigilance program:

1. **Regulatory knowledge:** Recognize the rules and regulations that apply to pharmacovigilance in your nation or area. This covers the need to comply with pertinent rules and regulations, identify signals, create risk management plans, and report unfavorable events.

2. **Dedicated team:** Assign the task of supervising and directing the program to a pharmacovigilance team. Pharmacovigilance specialists, medical doctors, data analysts, and regulatory affairs specialists could be on this team.

3. Establish detailed and unambiguous **standard operating procedures (SOPs)** that describe the methods for gathering, recording, evaluating, and reporting unfavorable events. Make sure that these processes adhere to the rules and regulations.

4. **Adverse Event reporting system:** Put in place a reliable system to gather and document reports of adverse events, this could be an electronic database or software intended for the effective collection, administration, and analysis of adverse event data.

5. **Education and training:** Educate employees engaged in pharmacovigilance on their roles and duties as well as the procedures for reporting and handling adverse events. It is crucial to receive ongoing training on modifications and advancements in pharmacovigilance procedures.

6. **Create risk management plans** for products that include methods for locating, reducing, and disclosing hazards related to pharmaceuticals. This entails carrying out risk analyses and putting risk reduction plans into action.

7. **Establish procedures for signal detection and analysis** in order to proactively spot any possible safety concerns related to prescription drugs. Data mining, trend analysis, and other techniques are used in this to find warning signs of unfavorable occurrences.

8. **Communication and reporting:** Create protocols to notify regulatory bodies of unfavorable events and to ensure that reporting

deadlines and specifications are met. It is essential to communicate both internally and internationally.

9. **Continuous improvement:** To find opportunities for improvement, regularly assess and audit the pharmacovigilance procedures, keep up with best practices, new advancements, and regulatory changes to make the program better all the time.

10. **Cooperation and networking:** Work together with other interested parties, including medical professionals, government organizations, and pharmacovigilance networks. Engaging in industry forums and exchanging experiences might yield significant insights.

11. **Compliance and audits:** To make sure that regulatory requirements and rules are being followed, conduct internal audits on a regular basis. Recognize any shortcomings and take appropriate corrective action.

12. **Periodic evaluations and documentation:** conduct regular evaluations of the pharmacovigilance data and keep a record of every action done, assessment completed, adverse event report, and other activity. To maintain the safety of pharmaceutical products, a strong pharmacovigilance program must be established. This involves taking a strategic approach, being committed to compliance, providing continual training, and focusing on continuous development, maintain thorough documentation for regulatory inspections and audits, establishing at a medical facility to guarantee patient safety and efficient tracking of adverse drug reactions (ADRs),

7.1. Pharmacovigilance programs must be established in hospital settings

The following is a customized method for doing so:

1. **Leadership and commitment:** Leadership Support: Obtain hospital administration approval to form a specialized pharmacovigilance team or assign current employees to do pharmacovigilance tasks.

2. **Education and Training:** Staff Training: Give all pertinent healthcare workers thorough instruction on pharmacovigilance principles, ADR reporting protocols, and the significance of documenting and reporting adverse events.

3. Establish standard operating procedures (SOPs): SOPs should be clear, succinct, and uniform in order to establish ADR reporting, documentation, and follow-up processes. Procedures for reporting and handling ADRs at the hospital should be outlined in SOPs.

4. ADR reporting system/ implemented reporting system: Provide a mechanism that enables medical personnel to quickly and conveniently report adverse drug reactions (ADRs). This mechanism may comprise electronic reporting forms or a dedicated reporting platform.

5. Cooperation and communication/ internal collaboration: To guarantee thorough ADR reporting and monitoring, promote cooperation and communication amongst many departments (pharmacy, nursing, and medical personnel).

6. Data collection and analysis/ ADR data collection: This involves the routine gathering and examination of ADR reports, along with the implementation of systems for examining and assessing them in order to spot patterns or any safety concerns.

7. Dedicated team or committee/ pharmacovigilance team: Form a team that will be in charge of analyzing ADR reports, carrying out evaluations, and putting risk-reduction plans into action.

8. Education Materials/Patient Education: Provide patients with informational materials about ADR reporting, urging them to notify medical professionals of any unexpected side effects from their medications.

9. Regulatory Compliance/ regulation adherence: Make sure that all local, state, and federal laws pertaining to pharmacovigilance and ADR reporting are followed.

10. Periodic review and improvement/ continuous improvement: Evaluate the pharmacovigilance program's efficacy on a regular basis. Make adjustments in response to criticism, data analysis, and new best practices.

11. Reporting and documentation: It keeps thorough records of all ADR reports, evaluations, and actions completed. Make sure that internal audits and regulatory compliance are properly documented.

12. Quality Assurance/ internal audits: Regularly carry out internal audits to assess the program's compliance and efficacy in pharmacovigilance. Recognize any shortcomings and put corrective measures in place.

7.2. Establishment & operation of drug safety department in industry:

To guarantee the efficacy and safety of pharmaceuticals, the pharmaceutical company must establish and run a drug safety department. Here are some crucial actions and things to think about:

Establishment:

Regulatory Understanding: Recognize and abide by the laws governing drug safety and pharmacovigilance (PV). Global regulations differ (for example, the US's FDA and Europe's EMA), so be sure you comply with all applicable authorities.

a. Hire a team of trained individuals with pharmacovigilance experience, such as doctors, pharmacists, nurses, and scientists who are experienced in reporting adverse events.
b. Infrastructure & Systems: Make a financial commitment to reliable systems for gathering, analyzing, and reporting data. This covers databases, signal detecting technologies, and safety management software.
c. Standard Operating Procedures (SOPs): Create thorough SOPs detailing the reporting, evaluation, communication, and detection of adverse events.
d. Training Programs: Ensure that staff members are informed about evolving technology, best practices, and regulatory changes by holding regular training sessions.
e. Operation: Adverse Event Reporting: Create protocols for gathering and evaluating adverse event reports from patients, healthcare professionals, publications, and clinical trials, among other sources.
f. Signal detection: Use signal detecting techniques to find patterns in unfavorable events or possible safety issues.
g. Create risk management plans, or RMPs, for high-risk pharmaceuticals. These documents should include strategies for reducing risks and keeping an eye on safety throughout the product's lifespan.
h. **PSURs, or Periodic Safety Update Reports:** At predetermined intervals, compile and submit PSURs to regulatory bodies that provide a summary of the safety profile of marketed medications.

Collaboration and communication are key to ensuring a coordinated approach to drug safety, encourage cooperation across several departments, including clinical, regulatory affairs, and marketing. Additionally, keep in touch with regulatory bodies about any modifications or safety issues.

i. **Continuous Improvement:** To meet changing regulatory requirements and boost the effectiveness of drug safety operations, routinely review and update procedures.

j. **Audits and inspections:** Keep correct records, follow SOPs, and make sure compliance to be ready for regulatory agency audits and inspections.

7.3. Contract Research Organizations (CROs)

CROs are businesses that offer a range of research services and support to the biotechnology, pharmaceutical, and medical device industries. They are vital to the development and testing of medications and medical products because they conduct clinical trials, research studies, and other services. An outline of CROs and their roles is provided below:

1. Clinical Research Organizations (CROs) provide services related to the management of clinical trials. These services include protocol preparation, patient recruiting, site management, data collection, and regulatory compliance.

2. Biostatistics and data management: They oversee the gathering, organizing, processing, and reporting of data during clinical trials, guaranteeing data accuracy and legal compliance.

3. Regulatory Affairs and Compliance: CROs offer proficiency in managing regulatory procedures, guaranteeing conformity to national and worldwide rules and directives.

4. Pharmacovigilance and Drug Safety: CROs manage risks associated with pharmaceutical goods and carry out pharmacovigilance tasks such as adverse event reporting and monitoring.

5. Medical Writing and Documentation: They create reports, clinical trial protocols, regulatory documents, and other vital paperwork needed to submit to regulatory bodies.

6. Assurance of Quality: CROs carry out evaluations and audits of quality assurance to make sure that regulations and Good Clinical Practice (GCP) guidelines are being followed.

Contributions and Roles:

a. Research support: CROs help pharmaceutical companies move their drug development pipeline forward by helping to plan and carry out research projects.

b. Efficiency and expertise: They provide resources and specialized knowledge, which frequently make it possible to conduct clinical trials and research more effectively and economically.

c. Risk mitigation: CROs assist in reducing risks by utilizing their systems, expertise, and experience to guarantee quality and compliance in research operations.

d. Flexibility and scalability: They provide pharmaceutical businesses with the capacity to access specialized services and resources in accordance with project requirements, owing to their flexibility and scalability.

Advantages of CRO Use:

1. Access to infrastructure and specialist knowledge without the requirement for substantial internal resources is known as specialized expertise.

2. Cost Efficiency: Solutions that are economical because they share resources and have reduced procedures.

3. Faster Timelines: By using their experience and effective administration, CROs can shorten the duration of research projects.

4. Decreased Risk: Help in negotiating intricate regulatory frameworks, which lowers the risk of noncompliance.

Aspects to consider when **working together** (In **Collaboration**):

a. Process of Selection: Pick a CRO according to their experience, reputation, standards of quality, and suitability for the project.

b. Communication and Cooperation: To guarantee project success, create explicit lines of communication and frameworks for cooperation.

c. Contractual Agreements: Create thorough contracts that specify duties, deadlines, deliverables, and agreements on confidentiality.

7.4. Creating a national program

Creating a national program in the healthcare system requires a thorough strategy, cooperation from a range of stakeholders, and a well-defined plan to accomplish particular health-related objectives. Here's how to set up a national health program, step-by-step:

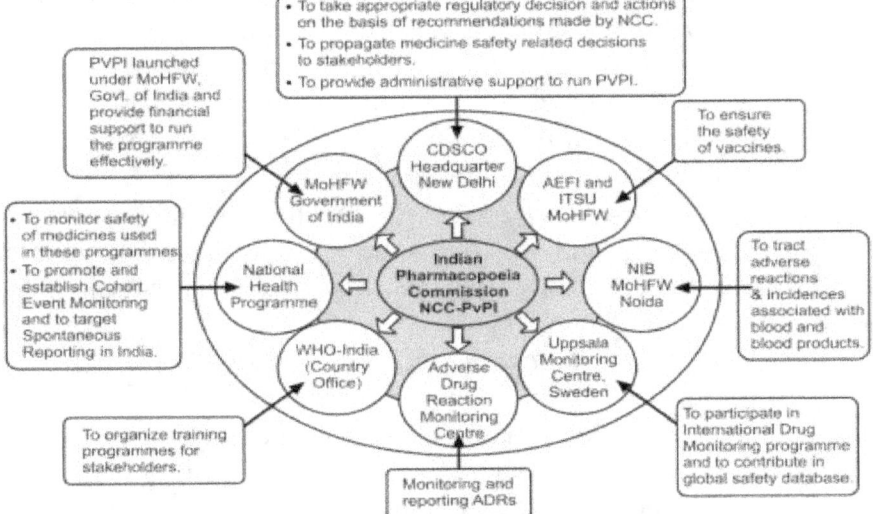

Fig. 4. National Healthcare Program

1. *Planning and needs assessment/ evaluate healthcare needs:* Determine the most important health challenges, top priorities, and service gaps by conducting a comprehensive evaluation of the nation's healthcare needs, establish specific goals: establish measurable goals for the national program that center on enhancing the availability of healthcare, the prevention or treatment of disease, or certain health outcomes.

2. *Collaboration and stakeholder engagement:* In order to obtain feedback and forge agreement, collaborate with governmental

organizations, healthcare providers, non-governmental organizations, patient advocacy groups, and other stakeholders, multi-sectoral collaboration: to address health factors holistically, form alliances between the health, education, finance, and social services sectors.

3. *Legislation and policy development:* Create guidelines and policies that specify the goals, tactics, and schedules for carrying out the national program, funding and legislation: obtain the necessary funds and legislative backing to ensure the program's implementation and long-term viability.

4. *Infrastructure and resources/ healthcare infrastructure:* Make the necessary investments in the facilities, machinery, technology, and infrastructure in the healthcare industry to meet the program's objectives, human resources: assure that healthcare professionals have the necessary training and staffing to carry out and oversee the program in an efficient manner.

5. *Phased implementation and monitoring:* Execute the program by dividing it into manageable chunks and making sure that each step is properly coordinated and monitored, monitoring and evaluation: provide systems, such as outcome measurements and key performance indicators (KPIs), for tracking and assessing the advancement of the program.

6. *Education and public awareness/ health promotion campaigns*: Start educating the public, medical professionals, and other stakeholders about the goals and advantages of the program, community engagement: involve local communities in initiatives to promote health and give them the tools they need to take an active role in the program.

7. *Data Collection and Analysis/Health Information Mechanisms:* Put in place reliable mechanisms for gathering data in order to monitor program outcomes, health indicators, and program effects, evidence-based decision making: make program modifications as needed, spot trends, and use data analysis to drive policy decisions.

8. *Iteration, adaptation, and continuous improvement:* Iterate, adapt, and evaluate the program's efficacy on a regular basis. Modify tactics in response to new information, knowledge sharing: disseminate best practices and lessons gained to other nations or areas dealing with comparable health issues.

9. Regulatory framework and compliance/ regulatory compliance: Throughout the program's execution, make sure that ethical standards, legal requirements, and global health conventions are followed, the establishment of a national health program necessitates the concerted effort, unwavering dedication, and cooperation of numerous stakeholders in order to address healthcare issues and enhance national health outcomes.

Unit 3

Chapter 8
Vaccine safety surveillance

A vital part of public health initiatives to prevent and control infectious illnesses is vaccine safety surveillance, it entails the ongoing evaluation and monitoring of vaccinations to guarantee their efficacy and safety following licensure and public introduction, finding and looking into any possible side effects linked to immunization is the main objective.

a. **Pre-licensure Clinical Trials:** A vaccine must pass these stringent testing procedures before being authorized for general use, thousands of people take part in these trials, which evaluate the vaccine's effectiveness, safety, and any side effects, regulatory approval is predicated on the evidence from these trials.

b. **Post-licensure surveillance:** After a vaccination is authorized and administered, continued observation is crucial, a number of mechanisms are in place to look into and identify adverse events that would not have been discovered in pre-licensure trials because of the small sample size or brevity of the studies,

c. **Passive surveillance**: The process of gathering unprompted reports of adverse events from the public, healthcare professionals, and vaccine makers is known as "passive surveillance" after receiving a vaccination, people have the option to voluntarily report any adverse events to various monitoring systems or national regulatory organizations.

d. **Active Surveillance:** This technique uses systematic data collecting to actively look for possible adverse events, to find any odd trends of adverse occurrences; this may entail keeping an eye on electronic health records, performing epidemiological research, and utilizing registries or databases.

e. **VAERS, or the Vaccine Adverse Event Reporting System**: It is a national system used in the United States to track vaccine safety. It is a passive surveillance system that depends on reports of adverse events following immunization from manufacturers, healthcare providers, and the general public.
f. **Worldwide Vaccine Safety Initiatives**: To create worldwide vaccine safety networks, nations partner with international organizations like the World Health Organization (WHO).
g. **Risk Communication:** It's essential to inform the public and medical professionals about the safety of vaccines in an effective manner building and sustaining confidence in immunization programs is facilitated by timely and transparent communication.
h. **Expert Committees:** Both domestic and foreign expert committees routinely examine safety data, evaluate possible hazards, and offer guidance to regulatory bodies and healthcare professionals.

8.1. Vaccine pharmacovigilance, often known as vaccine safety monitoring, is a subset of pharmacovigilance that focuses on identifying, evaluating, comprehending, and preventing vaccine-related side events and other issues.

a. Surveillance systems: It is essential to maintaining the safety of vaccines after they are administered, one of the fundamental elements of vaccine pharmacovigilance is the establishment and upkeep of surveillance systems to continuously monitor the safety of vaccinations. These systems could include active surveillance techniques like systematic data gathering from electronic health records or focused studies, as well as passive reporting systems where medical professionals and the general public voluntarily report adverse events.

b. Data collection and analysis: It is crucial to gather and examine information on adverse events that occur after vaccinations (AEFI). This covers not only severe or unanticipated side effects but also an examination of the background rates of typical health occurrences to look for any trends or patterns that may be connected to vaccination.

c. Risk assessment: Analyzing the advantages and disadvantages of vaccinations is a constant process. This entails weighing the advantages of vaccination, such as the avoidance of potentially serious or fatal infections, against the frequency and severity of adverse reactions.

d. Causality Assessment: A crucial component of vaccine pharmacovigilance is figuring out whether a reported adverse event is connected to immunization in a causal way. To prove or disprove a causal relationship, a variety of methods and instruments for assessing causality are employed.

e. Signal detection: Early action is dependent on the identification of signs indicating possible safety risks. This entails looking for any odd patterns or relationships that might require more research utilizing statistical approaches, data mining strategies, and other tools.

f. Creating and putting into practice **risk management plans**: To lessen hazards that have been recognized, such as revising product labels, changing immunization schedules, or adding more surveillance.

g. Reporting and communication: A crucial component of vaccine pharmacovigilance is informing medical professionals, government agencies, and the general public about vaccination safety information. Building and sustaining trust in immunization programs is facilitated by timely and transparent reporting.

h. Global collaboration: International cooperation is crucial since vaccination production and distribution are worldwide in scope. together, nations and organizations exchange information, knowledge, and best practices to improve vaccine safety on a global scale.

i. Post-Marketing Studies: Post-marketing studies are carried out to evaluate the long-term safety and efficacy of vaccines or to look at certain safety issues in more detail.

j. Regulatory Oversight: In order to ensure the safety of vaccines, regulatory bodies are essential. To guarantee the ongoing safety of vaccinations, they examine safety data, offer suggestions, and, if required, implement regulatory steps.

8.2. Vaccine failure:
When a person receives the required vaccination but does not experience the anticipated amount of immunity or protection against a particular disease, this is referred to as vaccination failure, although most people respond well to vaccines, not everyone gets 100% immunity from them.

Primary vaccine failure includes: Failure to receive vaccinations can have a number of causes, including:

1. Incomplete immune response: One of the main causes of vaccine failure is an insufficient immunological response. Some people might not respond to the vaccine well enough to provide adequate protection. Age, underlying medical issues, or a compromised immune system are a few examples of factors that may be involved.

2. Interference with other vaccines: When several vaccinations are given at the same time or very near to each other, the effectiveness of one or more of the shots may be diminished.

Secondary vaccine failure includes: Waning immunity is one type of secondary vaccine failure that can occur over time, certain vaccines can cause a reduction in the protective immunity they offer. For some vaccines, booster doses are advised in order to strengthen and extend immunity.

Emergence of new strains: The vaccine's efficacy against newly emerging strains may be diminished if the infectious agent (virus or bacteria) experiences genetic alterations. This is especially true for viruses such as the human immunodeficiency virus (HIV) and influenza.

Among the problems in administering and storing vaccines are:

1. Improper storage: To preserve their efficacy, vaccines must be kept in a particular temperature range. Vaccines may lose some of their effectiveness if they are stored or transported at incorrect temperatures.

2. Errors in vaccine administration: Using the incorrect dosage or delivery method, for example, can lessen the vaccine's efficacy.

Host variables consist of:

a. Immunocompromised people: Those with compromised immune systems, such as those receiving immunosuppressive therapies or suffering from certain illnesses like HIV/AIDS, may not react to vaccinations as well as they should.

b. Age-related factors: Compared to healthy adults, infants, the elderly, and people with immune system problems may not react to vaccinations as strongly. Not receiving all of the prescribed doses of a vaccine—certain vaccines need several doses to offer the best protection—is one example of an incomplete vaccination series. An individual might not fully develop immunity if they do not receive all of the prescribed vaccinations.

Challenges associated with vaccines include:

a. Vaccine Composition: Certain vaccines may not offer total protection against every pathogen strain due to their composition. For instance, not every strain of the flu may be protected against by the influenza vaccine.

b. Vaccine Variability: The effectiveness of vaccines may be impacted by manufacturing flaws or adjustments made to the production process. It's critical to remember that, even in situations where vaccinations don't work as intended, vaccinations are extremely vital for stopping the spread of dangerous diseases. When compared to unvaccinated individuals, the severity of the sickness and the risk of consequences are typically lower in those who receive vaccinations. In order to overcome vaccination failure, public health strategies—such as administering booster doses on a regular basis, keeping an eye on vaccine effectiveness, and modifying immunization plans in response to new patterns of infectious diseases—are crucial. Furthermore, continuous research and development work to advance vaccine technology and increase their efficacy.

8.3. Adverse Event Following Immunization (AEFI) are any unfavorable medical event that occurs after vaccination and is not always linked to the vaccine's administration. From minor, transient side effects to more severe or dangerous reactions, AEFIs can take many different forms. It's crucial to remember that most immunizations are safe and that severe side effects are uncommon. Typical and anticipated responses consist of:

a. Local reactions: Common and typically mild symptoms include pain, redness, or swelling at the injection site.

b. Systemic reactions: Fever, exhaustion, headaches, aches in the muscles, and moderate irritation are examples of systemic reactions. These are often transient and indicate that the body is fortifying its defenses.

Among the serious AEFIs are:

i. Anaphylaxis: An extreme allergic reaction known as anaphylaxis is an uncommon side effect of immunization. Although anaphylaxis is exceedingly rare, it does require immediate medical intervention.

ii. Guillain-Barré Syndrome (GBS): In extremely rare instances, a few vaccines have been linked to a higher chance of developing this neurological condition.

iii. Intussusception: A little elevated risk of intussusception, a form of intestinal obstruction, exists in relation to rotavirus vaccinations.

Monitoring and reporting AEFIs includes:

a. Vaccine Adverse Event Reporting Systems (VAERS): These systems, which are implemented in many nations, allow the public, healthcare professionals, and vaccine producers to record adverse events following vaccination. This data supports further surveillance of vaccination safety.

b. Surveillance Programs: To detect any possible safety issues, public health organizations keep a close eye on and look into complaints of adverse events. Figuring out causation is a part of the assessment of causality. It can be difficult to determine if a vaccination caused an adverse occurrence. In order to identify whether an adverse event is likely attributable to vaccination, health authorities employ specified criteria and instruments for causality assessment.

Risk-Benefit Analysis comprises the following:
a. Balancing benefits and risks: Generally speaking, the advantages of vaccination—such as preventing major diseases and associated complications—outweigh the chances of unfavorable outcomes. Health authorities evaluate and disseminate vaccinations' overall risk-benefit profile on a regular basis.

Included in education and communication are:
a. Open communication or Transparent communication: Establishing and preserving public confidence in immunization programs requires prompt and open information about possible risks and benefits.
b. Public education: Giving correct information about typical side effects and responding to concerns helps people make well-informed vaccination decisions.

Among the **preventive measures** are:
a. Screening for contraindications: In which medical professionals closely examine each patient to see whether they are a candidate for vaccination or have a history of serious allergic responses to vaccine ingredients.
b. Research on Vaccine Safety: Constant research endeavors to enhance vaccine safety and pinpoint methods to reduce unfavorable outcomes.

Chapter 9
Methods used in pharmacovigilance

The science and actions involved in the identification, evaluation, comprehension, and avoidance of side effects or any other issues relating to drugs are known as pharmacovigilance. Pharmacovigilance uses a range of techniques and instruments to guarantee the continued safety of pharmaceuticals, including vaccines, the following are some important pharmacovigilance techniques:

9.1. Passive surveillance: Spontaneous Reporting Systems:

a. Healthcare Professionals and Patients Reporting: This type of reporting, in which patients and healthcare professionals voluntarily notify regulatory bodies or pharmacovigilance centers about adverse drug reactions (ADRs), is the foundation of many pharmacovigilance systems.

b. Data mining is the process of using electronic health records and other healthcare databases to find possible indicators of unfavorable events, this is done using electronic health records (EHRs) and electronic medical records (EMRs). This entails analyzing huge databases for patterns or trends using statistical techniques.

c. Disease-Specific Registries: Keeping track of registries for certain diseases or conditions in order to keep an eye on the efficacy and safety of medications used to treat those disorders.

d. Vaccine Registries: Using specialized registries, vaccine safety and efficacy are tracked and monitored.

e. Identifying signals or signal detection:

1. Using statistical techniques to find any signs of disproportionate reporting that could point to a safety problem is known as quantitative signal detection.

2. Qualitative Signal Detection: To find possible signals, examine each case report in detail and look for trends or groups of unfavorable events.

Risk reduction methods are developed and put into practice as part of **risk management plans (RMPs)** in order to reduce known risks related to certain medications or vaccinations.

f. Communication Plans: Providing public and healthcare professionals with a framework for communicating in order to effectively disseminate safety information. Clinical Trials and Studies, conducted after marketing:

1. Pre-Marketing Clinical Trials: Before a medication or vaccine is licensed, extensive clinical trials are carried out to evaluate safety, effectiveness, and potential side effects.

2. Post-Marketing Surveillance Studies: tracking medications and vaccines after they are approved for use on the market in order to spot and assess uncommon or protracted side effects.

3. Conducting observational studies to evaluate the practical safety and efficacy of medications and vaccines in a range of populations is known as pharmacoepidemiology.

g. Review and Analysis of the Literature:

i. Systematic Literature Reviews: Analyzing published literature in-depth to learn about known and possible dangers associated with drugs.

ii. Combining and evaluating data from several trials to produce a more thorough evaluation of drug safety is known as meta-analysis.

iii. Cooperation and Information Sharing: International Cooperation: Working with institutions such as the International Council for Harmonization of Technical Requirements for Pharmaceuticals for Human Use (ICH) and the World Health Organization (WHO) to conduct international cooperation and information sharing.

Inspections and Audits of Pharmacovigilance:

a. Quality assurance involves carrying out audits and inspections to make sure that pharmacovigilance centers, regulatory bodies, and pharmaceutical corporations follow quality standards when gathering, reporting, and analyzing data.

b. By depending on spontaneous reports and case series provided by medical professionals, patients, or other sources, passive surveillance is a technique for keeping an eye on the safety of medications, vaccines, and other medical goods. It is a crucial part of pharmacovigilance, an effort to identify and evaluate unfavorable occurrences related to pharmacological interventions. This is a summary of passive surveillance that focuses on spontaneous reports and case series:

Definition of spontaneous reports: These reports are voluntary submissions of information to regulatory bodies or pharmacovigilance centers by patients, healthcare professionals, or other individuals regarding adverse events.

Information Source: Reports describing adverse responses seen following the administration of drugs or vaccines can be submitted by healthcare providers, individuals, and occasionally pharmaceutical firms.

Scope: Adverse occurrences ranging from common and moderate reactions to uncommon and major events might be included in spontaneous reports, a case series is a compilation of individual reports or cases of unfavorable occurrences connected to a specific medication or vaccination, these reports may be submitted by researchers, healthcare providers, or other sources.

Case Grouping: Similarity in the observed unfavorable events or the circumstances surrounding their occurrence is frequently used to group cases in a series.

Analysis: To find patterns, trends, or similarities among reported adverse occurrences, case series are examined. The benefits of passive surveillance include early signal identification, which makes it possible to identify possible safety issues in advance, particularly unusual or unanticipated adverse events.

Real-World Data: It offers information about vaccine and medication safety in the real world, away from the regulated setting of clinical trials.

Large-Scale Monitoring: Since many patients and healthcare professionals can submit reports, it enables large-scale population monitoring.

Problems and restrictions: Underreporting: Since not all adverse events are reported and because reporting rates can differ, underreporting is one of the main constraints.

Report quality: The capacity to do thorough analysis may be impacted by the differences in the completeness and quality of spontaneous reports.

Causality assessment: It can be difficult to establish a link between the reported adverse event and the medication or vaccination that was given.

Function in Pharmacovigilance: Complement to Other Methods: By offering a thorough grasp of medication safety, passive surveillance supports active surveillance and systematic literature studies, among other pharmacovigilance techniques.

Signal Generation: It plays a key role in identifying possible safety issues so that more research or legal action may be taken to address them.

Regulatory Reporting:

a. Mandatory Reporting: Pharmaceutical companies are mandated to notify regulatory authorities of specific adverse events in numerous countries, it may also be necessary or encouraged for patients and healthcare providers to report.

b. Regulatory Decision-Making: When deciding whether to update product information or put safety precautions in place, regulatory bodies consult data from spontaneous reports to ensure the ongoing safety of medications and vaccines.

9.2. Stimulated reporting:
Also referred to as solicited reporting, stimulated reporting is a pharmacovigilance technique in which medical practitioners proactively look for data on adverse events or side effects associated with the administration of drugs or vaccines, in contrast to spontaneous reporting, which occurs when individuals such as patients, healthcare professionals, or others voluntarily submit reports, stimulated reporting entails a more proactive approach to obtaining safety data, this approach is frequently used for certain medications or vaccines, or in particular circumstances.

The purpose of stimulated reporting is to proactively gather safety information, especially in instances where there may be specific concerns or a need for more comprehensive data on the safety profile of a drug or vaccination, these are some important points of stimulated reporting.

Settings for induced reporting:

a. Clinical Trials: Researcher information on adverse occurrences is actively sought after from study participants during clinical trials, this makes it possible to guarantee the quick detection and assessment of any possible safety concerns.

b. Post-Marketing Surveillance Studies: Following FDA approval and product launch, targeted studies aimed at gathering safety information from patients or healthcare professionals may be carried out to encourage reporting.

Stimulated Reporting Techniques:

1. Structured Questionnaires: To systematically gather data on adverse occurrences from patients or research participants, healthcare practitioners may employ structured questionnaires.

2. Surveillance Programs: To actively monitor a drug's or vaccine's safety, specific surveillance programs may be set up. To obtain information on safety, this may entail routine follow-ups with patients or healthcare professionals.

Advantages of Stimulated Reporting: Improved Data Collection: Stimulated reporting makes it possible to collect data in a more organized and methodical manner, making sure that certain negative events are actively sought out and documented.

Timely Identification of Safety Signals: Stimulated reporting can help with the timely identification of safety signals by actively gathering information, this can result in quicker responses and interventions when necessary.

Applications in Vaccine Safety Monitoring: Studies on Vaccine Safety: In the context of vaccinations, post-marketing studies may make use of stimulated reporting to actively gather safety information from immunized persons, particularly for novel or recently released vaccines.

Concerns or groups: Stimulated reporting may be used to track the safety of vaccines in certain groups, such as immunocompromised people or pregnant women, or where there are unique concerns regarding a given vaccine.

Regulatory Oversight:

Regulatory Requirements: As part of post-marketing obligations to guarantee a product's continued safety, regulatory bodies may in some circumstances force pharmaceutical companies to do stimulated reporting.

Risk Management Strategies: Plans for managing risks associated with specific medications or immunizations may include incentives for reporting.

9.3. Active surveillance: Drug event tracking, sentinel sites, and registries:

a. In pharmacovigilance, active surveillance entails proactively and methodically gathering information from patients, healthcare professionals, and other sources on adverse events or other safety-related matters, this technique differs from passive monitoring in that data is gathered voluntarily, active surveillance is very helpful in identifying uncommon or severe adverse events as well as in obtaining more thorough and trustworthy data. Three essential elements of active surveillance are as follows:

b. Sentinel sites are defined as certain medical facilities or geographic areas where ongoing surveillance of unfavorable incidents is carried out, these locations have been carefully picked to reflect a wider range of demographics.

The role of healthcare workers at sentinel sites in active surveillance involves the proactive reporting and monitoring of adverse events pertaining to medications or vaccinations. Using the gathered information, trends, patterns, or groups of unfavorable incidents can be found.

Definition of Drug Event Monitoring: Data on adverse events connected to a particular drug are systematically gathered and analyzed as part of this process, when a medicine is freshly introduced or has little safety information, this approach is frequently adopted.

Procedure: Patients or healthcare professionals are proactively approached and requested to report any unfavorable incidents they witness or encounter during medication use, this proactive strategy contributes to the prompt and thorough gathering of safety data.

Focus on Particular pharmaceuticals: Drug event monitoring may be started for particular pharmaceuticals of interest, particularly if their safety is under question or if they have just recently been released onto the market.

Registries: By definition, registries are structured databases that methodically gather and preserve data about people who have a specific illness, ailment, or have been exposed to a certain medication or vaccination. both passive and active forms of surveillance are possible with them.

Active Data Collection: Registries, when used in conjunction with active surveillance, entail actively contacting members of the registry in order to obtain information on treatment outcomes, adverse events, and other pertinent data.

Disease- or Product-Specific: Registries might be designed to track the safety and efficacy of a particular medication or vaccination, or they can be focused on people with a specific ailment.

Advantages of active surveillance: Prompt Adverse Event Identification: Prompt adverse event identification facilitates prompt responses and interventions.

Greater data comprehensiveness: Compared to passive surveillance, active surveillance techniques frequently produce more thorough and detailed data on unfavorable events since they are actively seeking out information.

Targeted surveillance: Targeted surveillance enables Targeted monitoring of safety risks by focusing on medications, vaccinations, populations, or geographic areas, the resource-intensive nature of active surveillance techniques presents certain challenges since they necessitate consistent efforts and resources to gather and examine data.

Limited Generalizability: Because data gathering is frequently targeted, conclusions drawn from active surveillance may not always apply to a larger population.

9.4. Comparative observational studies

9.4. Comparative observational studies: Which include cross-sectional, case control, and cohort studies, are research designs that compare various groups about a certain result of interest. Cross-sectional studies, case-control studies, and cohort studies are the three most popular forms of comparative observational research, every research design has advantages and disadvantages of its own.

These three categories are summarized as follows:

a. Cross-sectional study design: Data for a cross-sectional study are gathered all at once. Assessment of the exposure and result occurs concurrently.

Goal: Cross-sectional studies are helpful in characterizing the frequency of a specific condition or exposure in a population at a given moment in time.

Strengths: economical and speedy. beneficial for formulating theories. gives a glimpse of the population at a certain moment in time.

Cons: Inability to prove causation. doesn't include details regarding the chronological order of events. susceptible to bias in the event that exposure and outcome evaluation are conducted at different times.

b. Case-control study design: Studies using a case-control methodology are usually retrospective, they begin with people who have the desired outcome (cases) and people who do not (controls), next, the two groups' exposure histories are contrasted, the goal of case-control studies is to discover potential risk factors and to investigate uncommon diseases or outcomes.

Strengths: Effective in researching uncommon results. makes it possible to examine several exposures for a single result, can be completed more affordably and with comparable speed.

Limitations: susceptible to memory bias (different people may remember the same exposures), establishing temporal links is difficult, bias in selection if the controls don't accurately reflect the population.

c. Design of a Cohort Study: Cohort studies track a group of people throughout time according to their exposure status. The study's start determines the exposure, and participants are tracked to evaluate how the consequences have developed, the goal of cohort studies is to evaluate the causal relationship between exposures and outcomes, particularly in cases when the exposure is uncommon.

Strengths: Makes it possible to evaluate temporal causality. able to demonstrate a cause-and-effect connection, recall bias is less common than in case-control studies.

Cons: Could be costly and time-consuming, particularly for uncommon results, a lack of follow-up may result in bias, unfit for infrequent exposures.

The following are the main differences: Cross-sectional, simultaneous assessment, case-control, timing of exposure and result assessment. Exposure is evaluated retroactively after the event has happened.

Directionality: descriptive and cross-sectional; it does not prove causality or timing.

Case-Control: Retroactive; investigates the relationship between exposure and result.

Cohort: prospective; evaluates how exposure affects how outcomes evolve.

Cross-sectional: Effective and economical in terms of both efficiency and cost.

Case-Control: Relatively economical; more effective for uncommon outcomes.

Cohort: Could be costly and time-consuming, particularly in the case of uncommon results, participants are tracked prospectively after first exposure is established.

9.5. Targeted clinical investigations:

Research studies or trials that concentrate on particular facets, populations, or interventions in the field of clinical medicine are referred to as **targeted clinical investigations**, these studies are intended to answer particular queries or theories, and they are frequently directed by a focused strategy for acquiring pertinent data.

The following are some important details about targeted clinical investigations:

Focus areas: investigations that are specific to a particular disease or medical condition; these investigations may investigate aspects like etiology, pathophysiology, treatment modalities, or outcomes. studies that are Population-Specific: Certain studies may focus on particular populations, such as young patients, the elderly, or people with particular comorbidities.

Among the several kinds of targeted clinical investigations are interventional trials, which examine the results of a particular intervention—such as a novel medication, medical gadget, or therapeutic technique.

Studies that are observational in nature: These types of investigations focus on observing and analyzing particular features of an illness or condition without changing the course of treatment.

Objectives: Testing Hypotheses: In order to provide targeted solutions to the current questions, targeted investigations are frequently created to test particular hypotheses or research topics. Clinical outcomes include the effectiveness and safety of a treatment, the course of a disease, or the effect of a particular intervention on patient outcomes, clinical research can evaluate several kinds of clinical outcomes.

Patient Recruitment and Selection:

Inclusion and Exclusion Criteria: To specify the target population and guarantee homogeneity within the study group, studies usually have particular inclusion and exclusion criteria.

Stratification: To examine results within subgroups, researchers occasionally stratify the study population according to particular traits.

Phase III clinical trials are a type of targeted clinical investigation that involves conducting large-scale randomized controlled trials (RCTs) to evaluate the safety and effectiveness of novel interventions in comparison to established treatments.

Studies that analyze various treatment methods to ascertain which is most beneficial in actual clinical settings are known as Comparative Effectiveness Research, or CER.

Longitudinal Cohort Studies: observational research projects that track a cohort of participants across time to gather information on exposures, results, and possible confounding variables.

Regulatory Considerations: Approval and Oversight: To guarantee participant safety and ethical behavior, targeted clinical investigations—particularly interventional trials—frequently need regulatory approval and oversight from ethical review boards and regulatory bodies.

Data Analysis and Reporting:

Statistical approaches: To examine the gathered information and make inferences on the outcomes of interest, investigators employ statistical approaches.

Publication: The evidence basis in clinical medicine is bolstered by the dissemination of findings from focused clinical investigations through scientific publications.

Ethical considerations:

Informed Consent: In order to participate in targeted clinical investigations, participants must give informed consent that considers the goals, methods, possible hazards, and benefits of the study.

Ethical Review: To make sure the study protocol complies with ethical norms, institutional review boards (IRBs) or ethics committees examine and approve it.

Chapter 10
Communication in pharmacovigilance

10.1. Effective communication: It is essential to pharmacovigilance because it makes sure that all pertinent parties are aware of the safety profile of medications and medical supplies. Effective and punctual communication facilitates the identification, evaluation, comprehension, and mitigation of unfavorable consequences.

The following are important facets of pharmacovigilance communication:

a. Healthcare professionals reporting adverse occurrences: It is imperative to support and encourage healthcare professionals in reporting adverse occurrences in a timely manner, there should be clear reporting channels available, such as phone lines, online portals, and reporting forms.

Patients: Educating patients on the significance of informing their healthcare professionals or using approved channels of any unexpected or severe responses.

Regulatory authorities: It is imperative that pharmaceutical businesses and regulatory authorities communicate promptly, this include submitting other safety-related data as well as periodic safety update reports (PSURs), creating and disseminating risk management strategies is necessary to reduce hazards connected to certain medications or vaccinations.

1. Healthcare Provider Communication:

a. Product Information Updates: Using official channels and regulatory authorities, tell healthcare providers about updated product information, including safety alerts, warnings, and precautions.

b. Public Communication:

i. Public Announcements: Disseminating information about safety concerns or recalls via official channels, websites, and press releases.

ii. Guidelines and recommendations: Disseminating guidelines and recommendations for the use of particular drugs, particularly when safety concerns arise.

iii. Patient Information Leaflets: ensuring that information about possible hazards and adverse reactions is provided in an intelligible and straightforward manner in the patient information leaflets that come with drugs.

iv. Cooperation and Information Sharing: International Cooperation: Working together with regulatory bodies and international organizations to exchange safety information worldwide, participating in information-sharing platforms and pharmacovigilance networks in order to share information and insights.

v. Educational Initiatives: Educating for Healthcare Professionals: Educating and educating healthcare professionals on pharmacovigilance principles, risk management, and reporting obligations on an ongoing basis.

vi. Public Awareness Campaigns: Holding campaigns to inform patients about the value of reporting side effects and exercising caution when using medications.

2. Communication and Signal Detection:

a. Signal Communication: Promptly and openly informing pertinent parties about emergent safety signals.

b. Ensuring that the advantages and disadvantages of medications or vaccinations are conveyed in an impartial and clear way to facilitate well-informed decision-making is known as benefit-risk communication.

Creating and carrying out communication plans that specify methods for informing different stakeholders about safety information is one way to communicate risk.

Clear Messaging: Creating messages that are easy to read and comprehend in order to prevent misunderstandings and confusion regarding safety information, providing regular updates on the results of post-marketing surveillance studies and continuing safety monitoring initiatives is part of post-marketing surveillance.

Notifying pertinent parties of regulatory actions, such as label modifications, withdrawals, or limits, is known as "communication of regulatory actions."

c. Online reporting systems: Using online platforms to submit adverse event reports electronically is an example of electronic communication.

Web-Based Information Portals: Establishing web-based portals to provide the public and medical professionals with simple access to safety information, pharmacovigilance requires effective communication in order to ensure that information on the safety of medications and medical products is exchanged in a timely and transparent manner, many parties are involved in this communication, including patients, the public, pharmaceutical corporations, regulatory agencies, and healthcare professionals.

The following are fundamental ideas and tactics for accomplishing successful pharmacovigilance communication: avoid technical jargon, communicate in plain English, be transparent in your messaging, and utilize language that is easily understood by a wide range of people, including the general public and healthcare professionals. Be upfront and honest in your communication regarding the unknowns, constraints, and ongoing efforts to obtain further data, transparency helps stakeholders trust one another.

d. Reporting Adverse Events Promptly: Promote prompt reporting of adverse events by patients and healthcare workers.

Fast Dissemination: Make sure that pertinent stakeholders are informed as soon as possible about safety information, including updates, alerts, and warnings.

Regulatory Coordination:

Work Together with Regulatory Authorities: To exchange safety information and plan regulatory measures, establish efficient channels of contact with regulatory agencies. unified Messages: To prevent misunderstandings, make sure that safety messages from various regulatory bodies are consistent.

Healthcare Provider Engagement: Education and Training: Continually instruct medical professionals in risk communication, reporting guidelines, and pharmacovigilance principles.

Feedback systems: Provide systems that allow medical professionals to offer comments, pose inquiries, and look for answers to safety-related matters.

Patient empowerment: Inform patients about the significance of reporting adverse events and give them precise guidance on how to do so, this will increase patient engagement.

Patient information leaflets: Make sure that the patient information leaflets that come with prescription drugs include clear information about any possible dangers.

Cooperation with stakeholders: Industry Cooperation: Encourage pharmaceutical companies to collaborate in order to share safety data and plan joint risk management initiatives.

International cooperation: Take part in international cooperation to exchange safety information and coordinate worldwide pharmacovigilance initiatives.

Effective technology use: Online Platforms: Make use of online reporting platforms for adverse events to facilitate electronic report submission by patients and healthcare providers.

Web-Based information portals: Create web-based portals that give the public and medical professionals easy access to the most recent safety information.

Risk Communication Strategies:

Customized Messaging: Craft communications to appeal to certain target groups while taking their degree of medical expertise and information requirements into account.

Use of Visuals: To improve comprehension and memory of information, use infographics, visual aids, and other visual components.

Feedback Mechanisms:

Two-way contact: To get input from stakeholders and address their issues, set up two-way channels of contact. Reaction to Inquiries: Show your dedication to openness by providing prompt answers to questions and requests for information.

10.2. Crisis Communication Planning:

Readiness: Create and carry out crisis communication plans in order to effectively coordinate and communicate in the event of a growing issue or safety catastrophe.

Quick Reaction: Be ready to communicate clearly and quickly in the event of an emergency involving safety.

Adherence to Reporting Obligations: Comply with all applicable regulations on the reporting of adverse occurrences and the submission of safety data. When there are serious concerns about the safety of a medicine or medical product, communication is essential to addressing and resolving the situation, this is known as drug safety crisis management, during a crisis, efficient communication management promotes effective risk mitigation measures, accurate and timely information transmission, and the development and maintenance of stakeholder confidence.

The following are important guidelines and tactics for communication in drug safety crisis management:

Planning and readiness: create a thorough crisis communication plan ahead of time that specifies roles, duties, and communication procedures, establish clear channels of communication both within the company and with outside stakeholders, and designate important spokespersons.

Quick Reaction: As soon as there's a possible safety issue, get in touch, in order to answer public concerns and provide correct information, timeliness is essential, establish a round-the-clock communication system to react fast to new problems.

Transparency: Acknowledge any uncertainty and possible hazards in your communication about the situation, credibility and trust are increased by transparency, share with the public all that is known, the steps being taken to address the situation, and the investigations being conducted.

Consistent messaging: To prevent misunderstandings and preserve trust, make sure that communications are consistent throughout all communication venues, to guarantee that all parties involved receive regular updates, establish a single point of contact for information.

Communication focused on the audience: Customize communications for various groups of people, such as patients, healthcare providers, government regulators, and the general public, consider their comprehension levels and information needs, to improve comprehension, stay away from technical jargon and use simple language.

Multichannel Communication: To reach a variety of audiences, use a variety of communication channels, such as websites, social media, press releases, and traditional media, use technology, such as email alerts and cellphone notifications, to quickly disseminate information, engage with important stakeholders, such as industry partners, patient advocacy organizations, medical professionals, and regulatory bodies, create avenues of communication to get comments, answer questions, and give updates on the situation.

Training and Media Relations: Educate communication teams and spokespersons on message delivery, media relations tactics, and crisis communication techniques, in order to guarantee a cohesive and regulated message, establish media relations procedures and assign a spokesman.

Legal and Regulatory Compliance: Make sure that all communications adhere to legal standards and comply with regulatory obligations by working closely with legal and regulatory teams, recognize the legal ramifications of remarks you make in an emergency.

Constant Situation Monitoring and Updating: Keep an eye on things and notify relevant parties as soon as new information becomes available. Review the crisis communication plan frequently and modify tactics in light of the crisis' changing dynamics.

Post-Crisis Communication: After the crisis has been resolved, share information about the recovery efforts, remedial measures done, and lessons learned. Rebuild trust and reassure stakeholders of the safety precautions in place by maintaining constant communication.

10.3. Ethical Considerations: Prioritize patient safety and public health while upholding ethical norms in all communication initiatives. Refrain from downplaying dangers or making false claims that can undermine confidence. Interacting with Regulatory Authorities, Business Partners, Healthcare Facilities, and the Media: Pharmacovigilance and drug safety management require effective communication with regulatory agencies, business partners, healthcare facilities, and the media, every stakeholder group has different information demands, and good communication is crucial to upholding openness, guaranteeing compliance, and managing the pharmaceutical company's reputation, the following are important things to keep in mind when dealing with each stakeholder group:

a. Regulatory agencies: prompt reporting: adhere to regulations by providing accurate and timely reports on safety issues and adverse events, establish channels of open and cooperative communication with regulatory agencies in order to facilitate collaborative communication. Inform them of any updates to safety evaluations and risk reduction strategies.

Submission of Periodic Reports: In compliance with regulatory deadlines, submit the mandatory periodic safety reports, such as Periodic Safety Update Reports (PSURs) or Periodic Benefit-Risk Evaluation Reports (PBRERs).

Quick Response to Requests: Give regulatory authorities' requests for more details or clarification your full attention as soon as possible.

Business Partners: Proactive Communication: Address any safety concerns regarding joint ventures or products in a proactive manner with business partners. Establish channels for exchanging information between parties about safety updates, label modifications, and risk-reduction tactics.

Contractual Obligations: Observe the terms of the contract with regard to reporting safety incidents and corresponding with business associates.

Healthcare Facilities and personnel: Educational Initiatives: Educate healthcare personnel about product safety, possible dangers, and adverse event reporting procedures through educational materials and training sessions.

Clinical Updates: To guarantee educated prescription practices, healthcare institutions should be updated about pertinent clinical updates, safety alerts, and modifications to product information.

Reaction to Inquiries: Provide accurate and current information on product safety in response to questions from healthcare professionals as soon as possible.

Media: Proactive Communication: When there are major safety-related incidents or safety crises, communicate with the media in a proactive manner. A qualified spokesperson should be assigned to deal with the media on behalf of the organization, guaranteeing precision and coherence in the message.

Press Releases and Briefings: To ensure accurate information is distributed, release press releases on schedule and with transparency, hold press briefings, and use a variety of media outlets.

Crisis Communication strategy: During unfavorable occurrences, have a clear strategy in place that outlines important actions, roles, and communication techniques.

Patients and the Public: Patient Information Leaflets: Make sure that the information on possible dangers, adverse reactions, and reporting procedures is presented in an easy-to-read manner in patient information leaflets.

Public Awareness Campaigns: Inform patients about the significance of reporting adverse events and the appropriate channels for doing so by holding public awareness campaigns.

Online Platforms: Use social media and the firm website, among other online platforms, to give the public accurate and easily available safety information, coherent communication strategies are ensured by facilitating cross-functional collaboration amongst many departments within the firm, including pharmacovigilance, regulatory affairs, legal, and marketing.

Internal Training: To guarantee a consistent approach, provide internal training on pharmacovigilance concepts and the company's communication policy.

Messaging Consistency: unified messages: To prevent misunderstandings and preserve credibility, make sure safety messages are consistent throughout all communication channels.

Alignment with Labeling Changes: Coordinate any labeling modifications or risk-reduction strategies with external communications.

Legal Review: Examine all external communications for compliance with regulatory standards, legal considerations, and ways to reduce legal risks.

Prevent False Claims: Refrain from downplaying or making false claims that could result in legal repercussions.

Continuous Evaluation and Monitoring: Monitoring Effectiveness: Evaluate and monitor communication tactics on a regular basis, adjust in response to stakeholder reactions, comments, and new safety information.

Post-catastrophe Evaluation: To pinpoint lessons learned and opportunities for development, conduct a comprehensive assessment of communication activities following a catastrophe.

Unit 4

Chapter 11
Generating safety data

Generating safety data: The methodical process of gathering, examining, and evaluating data to determine the safety profile of medications, immunizations, medical equipment, and other healthcare interventions is known as safety data creation. This procedure is a key part of pharmacovigilance, which seeks to recognize and comprehend dangers and unfavourable events related to medicinal products at every stage of their lifecycle. The key elements of producing safety data are as follows:

a. Clinical Examinations:
i. Pre-approval Phase: Before a product is given regulatory approval, safety data is produced during clinical studies.
ii. Clinical trial phases: Phase IV involves post-approval surveillance, while Phases I through III examine dose, safety, and effectiveness in human subjects.
iii. Adverse Event Reporting: Serious adverse events (SAEs) and adverse events (AEs) are systematically reported during clinical studies.
iv. Post-Marketing monitoring reporting adverse occurrences voluntarily: Medical practitioners and patients may choose to notify pharmaceutical firms or regulatory bodies of adverse occurrences.
v. Passive Surveillance Systems: Data on safety from a variety of sources can be gathered more easily with the help of spontaneous reporting systems like the Vaccine Adverse Event Reporting System (VAERS).
vi. Signal Detection: Data that is spontaneously reported can be analysed to identify possible safety signals that may need more research.

b. Monitoring in Action:

i. Prospective Studies: To actively track safety results in real-world situations, prospective observational studies are carried out, such as cohort studies or registries.

ii. Targeted surveillance programs: Starting Targeted surveillance programs, particularly when safety issues emerge, for certain people or products.

iii. EHRs, or electronic health records, and RWD, or real-world data: EHR Integration: The process of extracting safety information from regular clinical practice by using electronic health records.

iv. Real-World Evidence (RWE): Data from real-world analyses are analysed to produce proof of the safety of medical goods across a range of patient demographics.

c. Sources of Pharmacovigilance Data:

i. Global Databases: For thorough safety data, use international pharmacovigilance databases, such as the WHO Global Individual Case Safety Reports (ICSRs) database.

ii. Aggregate Analysis: Analysing safety data in aggregate to find patterns and trends.

iii. Risk Assessment and Mitigation Techniques (REMS):

Implementation: To guarantee safe use, REMS programs should be put in place for certain medications that have known or possible major risks.

Assessment: Ongoing assessment of REMS programs' efficiency in reducing risks and enhancing product safety.

d. Systematic Reviews and Literature Reviews:

i. Systematic literature reviews: Compiling facts and data on safety by conducting systematic reviews of the scientific literature.

ii. Conducting meta-analyses is a method of synthesizing safety results from several studies.

iii. Clinical Results Evaluations: Using patient-reported outcomes (PROs) allows researchers to better understand how patients feel about safety outcomes.

iv. Measures of Quality of Life: Evaluating how medical products affect patients' overall well-being, both physically and mentally.

e. Biomarkers and biorepositories:
i. Biorepositories: Gathering biological material to enable medication safety research using genetics and biomarkers.
Analysing biomarkers linked to safety outcomes in order to pinpoint possible dangers or risk factors is known as biomarker analysis.

f. Plans for Risk Management (RMPs):
i. Pre-approval Planning: Creating RMPs to specify risk monitoring and mitigation techniques throughout the pre-approval stage.
ii. Post-Marketing Updates: Modifying RMPs in response to changing safety data and legal mandates.
iii. International Cooperation:
International Collaboration: Working together to exchange safety information and insights with international organizations, industry partners, and international regulatory bodies.
Harmonization of Standards: Helping to bring safety standards and procedures into line in order to make data generation more uniform, the process of creating safety data is continuous and involves a number of parties, including patients, healthcare providers, regulatory agencies, and pharmaceutical corporations. The incorporation of diverse data sources and approaches augments the comprehensive comprehension of medical product safety profiles, hence aiding in well-informed decision-making and safeguarding public health.

11.1. Preclinical phase: Prior to a possible new drug or medical product being tested on humans, the preclinical phase is the first step in drug development. In order to evaluate the experimental compound's pharmacological characteristics, safety, and effectiveness, laboratory and animal experiments are conducted at this phase. Preclinical phase goals include identifying potential safety concerns and collecting critical data to bolster the case for advancing a medication candidate into clinical trials. The following are significant preclinical phase elements:

Finding and Identifying the Target:

i. Finding a therapeutic target: Scientists pinpoint a particular molecular or biological target connected to a certain illness or condition.

ii. Lead compound identification: This procedure entails figuring out which chemical compounds are capable of interacting with the target.

iii. Research in vitro:

a. Cell culture experiments: Examining in controlled lab environments how the lead ingredient affects cells, analysing a compound's interactions with biological systems and comprehending its absorption, distribution, metabolism, and excretion (ADME) features are known as pharmacodynamics and pharmacokinetics.

b. In Vivo investigations on animals:

Acute Toxicity Studies: Evaluating the compound's direct harmful effects at various dosages.

Sub-chronic and chronic toxicity studies: Examining toxic effects that last for several weeks or months, analysing the behaviour of the substance in living things is known as pharmacokinetics and pharmacodynamics in animals.

iv. Investigative toxicology research:

Genotoxicity studies: Evaluating the compound's ability to cause genetic harm.

Studies on carcinogenicity: Examining if a substance has the capacity to cause cancer.

Studies on dose-response: Determining the range of doses that have therapeutic effects without producing appreciable harm is known as "establishing safe doses" identifying the buffer between harmful and effective doses is part of the process of defining the therapeutic window.

Creation and distribution: Formulation optimization refers to creating a formulation that makes it possible to administer the substance in a way that is both safe and efficient.

Choosing the administration route: Choosing the oral, intravenous, or other administration route that will most effectively deliver the substance to the intended target.

Planning and regulatory interaction:
Communication with regulatory bodies: Discussion of the suggested development strategy and resolution of any issues with regulatory bodies.
Pre-IND (Investigational New Drug) meetings: gatherings with regulatory bodies to talk about strategies for advancing into clinical trials and preclinical findings.

IND-supporting research:
Ensuring that preclinical research is carried out in accordance with GLP regulations is known as good laboratory practice, or GLP.
IND submission: Getting ready to submit an IND application to the appropriate regulatory bodies.

Moral aspects to consider:
Animal welfare: Using animals for research while upholding moral standards.
Reducing animal use: Using techniques to reduce the quantity of animals utilized while still gathering valuable information.

Reporting and Data Analysis:
Data interpretation is the process of evaluating preclinical data to determine the compound's safety, toxicity, and effectiveness.
Study Reports: Drafting comprehensive preclinical study reports for internal and regulatory filing, the basis for moving a medication candidate into clinical trials is the successful conclusion of the preclinical stage, before subjecting humans to experimental interventions, choices on the safety and possible efficacy of the investigational product must be made based on the evidence collected during this phase.

11.2. Phases of clinical trial:
Testing a novel medication or medical intervention on human volunteers to determine its safety and effectiveness is the clinical phase of drug development. Phase I,

Phase II, and Phase III are the divisions of this phase, and each includes a growing number of participants and distinct goals. Obtaining detailed information about the drug's safety profile, dose range, possible side effects, and efficacy in treating the intended ailment is the main objective. The following are the salient features of every stage in the clinical development process:

Phase 0: Investigative Experiments (Exploratory phase)
The phrase "phase zero" is not a standard phase in the usual clinical trial phases (Phase I, II, III, and IV), though it is sometimes used to describe **exploratory**, pre-phase I studies. The goal of these small-scale investigations is to gather basic information about a drug candidate's pharmacokinetics and pharmacodynamics.
Goal: Assess the drug's pharmacokinetics (PK) to learn how the body metabolizes, excretes, distributes, and absorbs the medication.
Analyze drug pharmacodynamics (PD): Look at the effects of the drug on the body, including any potential biomarkers and the mechanism of action.
Evaluate the Potential for Further Development: Help scientists decide whether to proceed with traditional phase I trials or to modify the drug candidate before further development, micro-doses, or extremely small doses, of the investigational medicine are commonly used in phase zero studies to minimize any potential risks to research participants. These studies are particularly useful when doing standard phase I investigations may not be feasible or when preliminary data is required to guide further study, it's crucial to keep in mind that not all situations and locations will accept or utilize the term "phase zero" in the same way. Periodically, it can refer to early exploratory studies carried out before to phase I trials. Researchers and regulatory bodies may employ different classification and nomenclature systems. Always refer to the exact guidelines and criteria provided by the regulatory agencies in charge of overseeing clinical trials in a particular field.

Phase I: Dosage and Safety
Goal: Evaluate the investigational drug's safety and dosage range.
Participants: Consists of a small number of people with the target disease or healthy volunteers.

Important Tasks: Analyze the pharmacokinetics, safety, and tolerability of the medication.
Establish the proper range of dosages.
Determine any possible negative reactions and side effects.
Evaluate the initial effectiveness, if relevant.

Phase II: Indications and Adverse Reactions
Goal: Examine the medication's effectiveness and continue to evaluate its safety.
Participants: This enrolls a greater number of people suffering from the intended illness.
Important Tasks:
Evaluate the medication's ability to treat the ailment.
Collect more safety information from a greater number of patients.
Examine the best dosages to achieve therapeutic effects.
Keep an eye out for and report unfavorable incidents.

Phase III: Trials of Confirmation:
Goal: Verify the medication's safety and effectiveness with a broader range of patients.
Participants Consists of a wider range of patients suffering from the intended illness.
Important Tasks:
Continue to assess safety and efficacy in regulated environments.
Gather information about uncommon negative consequences or incidents.
Verify the recommended dosage.
Provide information in submissions for regulatory approval.

Submission of Regulations:
Data Compilation: Gather extensive information from clinical and preclinical research.
Regulatory Submissions: Submit applications (such as the New Drug Application or the Biologics License Application) for regulatory approval.
Regulatory Review: To evaluate the overall risk-benefit profile, safety, and effectiveness, regulatory bodies examine the data that has been presented.

Phase IV: Post-Approval Monitoring

Goal: After receiving regulatory approval, carry out ongoing safety and efficacy monitoring of the medication.

Participants: During the post-marketing stage, a broader patient population is involved.

Important Tasks:

Keep an eye on long-term security in an actual environment.

Evaluate the medication's effectiveness in a range of patient demographics.

Identify and take care of any safety issues that were overlooked before.

Phase Sub-Phases IIA, IIB, and IIIB:

Goals: Optimize dosage, investigate new indications, or collect more detailed information.

Participants: May focus on particular subgroups or investigate various facets of drug usage.

Important Tasks:

Adjust dosing schedules.

Examine the medication's effectiveness in particular patient populations.

Answer any queries that remain from earlier stages.

Increased Access Initiatives:

Goal: Give patients who are not eligible for clinical trials yet have severe or life-threatening illnesses access to experimental medications.

Participants: People who fit certain requirements.

Important Tasks:

Attend to the unmet medical requirements of patient groups.

Get more information on safety and effectiveness.

Encourage the drug's compassionate use.

Phase 0: Investigative Experiments

Goal: Gather preliminary information to evaluate the drug's behavior in humans prior to moving forward with conventional Phase I studies.

Participants: Only a very limited number of subjects are involved.

Important Tasks:
Get a basic understanding of the pharmacokinetics and pharmacodynamics of the medication.

In order to evaluate early human metabolism, micro dosing might be used.

Patient safety, regulatory compliance, and adherence to ethical principles are critical throughout the clinical development phase. The outcomes of these stages have an impact on decisions regarding the drug's approval, labelling, and application in clinical practice. A new therapy's ability to treat patients depends on the successful completion of each phase of the clinical development process, which is a difficult and resource-intensive undertaking.

11.3. Post Marketing Surveillance (PMS):

Once a medication or medical product has received regulatory approval and entered the market, the post-approval phase, also known as Phase IV or Post-Marketing Surveillance (PMS), begins. This stage is essential for continuing to assess the product's efficacy and safety in real-world situations. The objectives of post-approval efforts are to maximize the usage of the product in a variety of patient categories, assess long-term safety and efficacy, and detect and manage any new or uncommon adverse events. Key elements of the post-approval stage are as follows:

Monitoring Unfavourable Events:
Systems for Spontaneous Reporting: Keep an eye on and evaluate reports of unplanned adverse events that patients, healthcare providers, and other sources submit.

Pharmacovigilance Databases: Use pharmacovigilance databases to continuously compile and examine safety data.

Signal Identification and Assessment:
Signal Detection: To identify possible safety signals that might point to hazards or patterns that have not yet been identified, apply statistical and analytical techniques.

Risk Management Techniques: If new safety issues are found, put risk management techniques into practice.

Risk-benefit analysis:
On the basis of actual facts, continuously evaluate the product's overall risk-benefit profile.
Risk and Benefit Balancing: Consider the trade-offs between established advantages and possible disadvantages for various patient populations.

Updates on Labelling and Communication:
Modifications to Labelling: Revise product labels to include updated safety data, modified dosages, and other pertinent information.
Communication with Healthcare Professionals: Use electronic communication channels, educational materials, and Dear Healthcare Professional letters to provide healthcare professionals with up-to-date safety information.

Pharmacoeconomic Research:
Determining Cost-Effectiveness: Perform pharmacoeconomic analyses to determine the product's cost-effectiveness relative to other available therapies.
Real-World Results: Examine the product's financial impact in actual clinical settings.

Retrospective Clinical Trials:
Confirmatory Studies: Post-marketing clinical trials should be carried out to address particular concerns about safety, effectiveness, or use in particular groups.
Long-Term Safety: Look into the long-term efficacy and safety of the product.

Studies on Paediatric and Special Populations:
Paediatric Research: To confirm the product's safety and effectiveness in paediatric populations, do paediatric research.
Studies on Special Populations: Examine how the product is used in groups with particular needs, such as the elderly or people with particular comorbidities.

Risk Assessment and Mitigation Techniques (REMS):
Continuous Evaluation: Evaluate any REMS programs that were put in place during the pre-approval stage on a regular basis.
Adjust REMS tactics as necessary in light of continuing safety evaluations.

Post-Marketing Monitoring in Foreign Nations:
International Cooperation: Work together with regulatory bodies in other nations to exchange safety data and carry out worldwide post-marketing surveillance.
Harmonization of Data: Help bring post-marketing surveillance standards and procedures into uniformity.

Patient Databases:
Establishment: Set up patient registries to monitor the product's long-term effects and users' safety.
Real-World Evidence (RWE): Make decisions based on real-world information gleaned from registries.

Evaluations of Health Technology:
Evaluating health impact: Examine the product's overall effects on health, considering how it affects patient outcomes, the use of healthcare resources, and public health.

Interaction with Patients:
Patient education: Continually instruct patients on how to utilize the product in a safe and efficient manner.
Patient Information Materials: Create and disseminate educational resources to help patients better grasp the advantages and disadvantages of various treatments.

Audits and Inspections for Pharmacovigilance:
Internal audits: Perform internal audits to make sure that post-marketing surveillance and pharmacovigilance regulations are being followed.
Regulatory Inspections: Get ready for and handle pharmacovigilance-related regulatory inspections.

The post-approval stage is essential for preserving the harmony between a marketed product's benefit and danger. To guarantee that any new safety issues are handled quickly and that patients and medical professionals have access to the most recent information, it entails ongoing monitoring, assessment, and communication. Throughout the post-approval stage of pharmacovigilance, patients, healthcare providers, pharmaceutical companies, and regulatory authorities all have significant responsibilities to play.

Chapter 12
ICH Pharmacovigilance Guidelines

ICH Pharmacovigilance Guidelines: The International Council for Harmonization of Technical Requirements for Pharmaceuticals for Human Use (ICH) has published guidelines for standardizing and harmonizing drug development methods, including pharmacovigilance. A framework for guaranteeing the safety of pharmaceutical goods throughout their entire lifecycle is provided by these standards. Relevant to pharmacovigilance are the following important ICH guidelines:

ICH E2A: Standards and Definitions for Accelerated Reporting in Clinical Safety Data Management: Establishes guidelines and terminology for the accelerated submission of individual case safety reports (ICSRs) during the medication development process.
lays out the standards for judging if a negative incident qualifies as "expedited."

ICH E2B: Clinical Safety Data Management: Information Needed to Send Specific Case Safety Reports: Outlines the information components that must be sent with ICSRs between pharmaceutical companies and regulatory bodies.
specifies the format and organization for safety data transfer via electronic means.

ICH E2C: Clinical Safety Data Management: Regular Safety Update Reports for Medicinal Products: Offers instructions for creating Periodic Safety Update Reports (PSURs) for medications that are already on the market, describes the structure and content of PSURs, including benefit-risk analyses and safety data.

ICH E2D: Standards and Definitions for Accelerated Reporting in Post-Approval Safety Data Management: Carries over the ICH E2A guidelines into the post-approval stage, stressing the significance of prompt safety information reporting.

ICH E2E: Planning for Pharmacovigilance: Offers direction on how to organize and carry out pharmacovigilance operations at every stage of a drug's lifespan, describes factors to consider while creating a pharmacovigilance plan, including risk control and communication tactics.

ICH E2F: DSUR (Development Safety Update Report): Explains the idea behind the Development Safety Update Report (DSUR), a document that compiles safety data while a clinical study is being conducted, aims to expedite the investigational phase's safety reporting requirements.

ICH E4: Information on Dose-Response for Drug Registration Support: Offers direction on how to gather and evaluate dose-response data while developing new medications, highlights how crucial it is to comprehend how drug exposure and reaction are related, taking safety precautions into account.

ICH E6: Integrative Added Note to ICH E6(R1) on Good Clinical Practice (GCP): Focuses on using best practices for clinical trials in terms of planning, carrying out, documenting, and reporting, highlights the significance of safety reporting and monitoring in relation to clinical studies.

ICH E9: Statistical Guidelines for Clinical Trials: Offers direction on statistical concepts for clinical trial design, conduct, analysis, and interpretation, incorporates safety assessment factors and statistical methods for managing safety data.

ICH E19: Safety Data Collection Optimization: Offers recommendations for improving the gathering of safety data during clinical trials in order to improve risk assessment and signal detection, highlights how crucial it is to use suitable safety data collection techniques, by simplifying the exchange of safety information and guaranteeing a uniform approach to safety monitoring throughout the medication development process and post-marketing period, these ICH guidelines aid in the global harmonization of pharmacovigilance methods. To ensure the safety of pharmaceuticals, it is critical that pharmaceutical companies, regulatory bodies, and other relevant parties are aware of and follow these rules.

12.1. ICH's goals and organization:
An international organization called the International Council for Harmonization of Technical Requirements for Pharmaceuticals for Human Use (ICH) unites regulatory bodies with the pharmaceutical sector to create and standardize guidelines and standards pertaining to the creation, registration, and post-approval of pharmaceutical products. The main goals of ICH are to improve public health, ease international trade, and encourage the efficacy and efficiency of drug research and registration processes. An outline of the company and its goals is provided below:

The ICH is organized as follows:
a. Participants: ICH is a special organization that brings together the pharmaceutical sector and regulatory bodies. Members include business associations such as the International Federation of Pharmaceutical Manufacturers and Associations (IFPMA) and regulatory bodies from various regions, including the European Union (EMA), Japan (PMDA), and the United States (FDA).

b. Groups of experts working (EWGs): Expert Working Groups (EWGs) within ICH are dedicated to particular areas of pharmaceutical development or issues of interest. Experts from industry and regulatory bodies make up these organizations.

c. Committee for steering: The ICH Steering Committee is in charge of supervising the organization's operations. It consists of members from industry and regulatory bodies who give the working groups guidance and leadership.

ICH's goals are as follows:
1. Harmonization: The aim is to avoid duplication of effort and promote worldwide development by harmonizing technical standards for pharmaceutical product development, registration, and post-approval.

Benefits: By streamlining the medication development process, harmonization enables regulatory decisions to be made in many locations more quickly and uniformly.

2. Improvement of Safety and Efficacy:

Goal: By creating standardized scientific methods and standards, we can improve technical and scientific knowledge of product safety and efficacy.

Benefits: A deeper comprehension of safety and efficacy enables the creation of pharmaceuticals that are both safer and more effective.

3. Global Registration Assisted:

Goal: Make it easier for regulatory applications to be accepted across different jurisdictions, allowing for quicker and more effective worldwide pharmaceutical product registration.

Benefits: Early patient access to safe and innovative medications is made possible by accelerated worldwide registration timelines.

4. Optimization of Resources:

Goal: Reduce needless duplication of work in the creation and evaluation of pharmaceutical products in order to maximize resource utilization both inside regulatory bodies and the pharmaceutical sector.

Benefits: Regulatory bodies and industry stakeholders gain from resource optimization's reduced costs and increased efficiency.

5. Following Approval Actions:

Goal: Address problems and obstacles that arise after approval, such as continuous safety monitoring and the creation of post-approval modification procedures.

Benefits: Ongoing cooperation guarantees the resolution of post-approval issues, enhancing the safety and efficacy of products.

6. Worldwide Public Health:

Goal: Advance the creation of safe, effective, and high-quality pharmaceutical products in order to improve public health worldwide.

Benefits: Improving public health outcomes is facilitated by guaranteeing that safe and effective medications are available everywhere.

7. Global Collaboration:
Goal: Promote global cooperation and coordination between the pharmaceutical industry and regulatory bodies.
Benefits: Cooperation leads to reciprocal acknowledgment of regulatory decisions and a shared awareness of global regulatory expectations.

8. Education and Developing Capabilities:
Goal: Encourage efforts aimed at strengthening capacity and enhancing regulatory knowledge and comprehension of ICH principles through training.
Benefits: Increasing regulatory capability contributes to the successful national adoption of harmonized norms, all things considered, ICH is essential to the advancement of pharmaceutical development worldwide because it provides a forum for cooperation and harmonization, which eventually helps patients, authorities, and the pharmaceutical sector, the organization works to ensure that high-quality medications are efficiently and promptly available to everyone on the planet.

Quick reporting: Within the field of pharmacovigilance, expedited reporting pertains to the prompt and efficient submission of safety data, specifically related to adverse events or potential adverse responses, to regulatory bodies at the development and post-commercialization stages of a pharmaceutical or medical device. The purpose of expedited reporting is to quickly disseminate critical safety information that could affect a medication's benefit-risk profile. Important features of reporting more quickly include:

a. Reports on Individual Case Safety (ICSRs):
Definition: A report containing details on one or more adverse events connected to the administration of a medication is known as an Individual Case Safety Report (ICSR).

12.2. Expedited Reporting:

12.2. Expedited Reporting: A few unfavourable events must be notified to regulatory agencies within a certain amount of time in order to be covered by expedited reporting.

ii. Accelerated Reporting Standards:

Seriousness: Incidents that are regarded serious and frequently call for prompt reporting include those that are lethal, seriously ill, hospitalized, result in long-term or major disability or incapacity, or cause congenital abnormalities or birth defects.

Unexpectedness: Events that could affect the product's risk-benefit ratio or that are unexpected given the drug's established safety profile may need to be reported more quickly.

Schedules for Accelerated Reporting:

Development Phase: Depending on the severity and conditions, sponsors may be obliged to disclose certain serious and unexpected adverse events within a short period of time (e.g., 7 or 15 calendar days) during clinical development.

Post-Marketing Phase: Reporting requirements for faster deadlines for serious and unforeseen incidents can vary, but they often call for reporting within 15 days.

Legal prerequisites: The International Council for Harmonization of Technical Requirements for Pharmaceuticals for Human Use (ICH) has established recommendations, specifically ICH E2A and ICH E2D, which offer direction on expedited reporting in the post-approval and clinical development stages.

Local Regulatory Requirements: Sponsors must abide by the laws of the areas where their goods are approved or being developed, and national regulatory bodies may have particular requirements for rapid reporting.

Quick Reporting Procedures:

Safety Databases: In order to gather and organize safety data, including adverse events, sponsors keep up safety databases, pharmacovigilance activities and safety databases differ slightly between countries due to differences in healthcare systems, regulatory frameworks, and reporting requirements. The safety database management processes used in pharmacovigilance for a few key categories are briefly summarized here:

a. US (FDA, or Food and Drug Administration): In the US, pharmacovigilance activities are overseen by the FDA, the primary safety database, the FDA Adverse Event Reporting System (FAERS), allows patients, healthcare providers, and manufacturers to record adverse events related to drugs and other medical supplies, FDA-mandated summaries of safety data for pharmaceutical companies' marketed drugs are known as periodic safety reports, or PSRs.

b. The European Union's European Medicines Agency (EMA): The EMA is in charge of organizing pharmacovigilance initiatives inside the European Union (EU), the EudraVigilance database, which serves as a centralized hub for compiling and assessing individual case safety reports (ICSRs), is managed by the European Medicines Agency (EMA).

c. Marketing authorization holders (MAHs): Operating in the EU are required to submit periodic safety update reports, or PSURs, to regulatory organizations.

d. The Japanese Pharmaceutical and Medical Devices Agency (PMDA): In Japan, pharmacovigilance operations are overseen by the PMDA. The Japanese Adverse Drug Event Report (JADER) database is used to collect and evaluate adverse event reports, similar to other countries, marketing permission holders in Japan are required to submit regular safety reports.

e. Health Canada, Canada: Pharmacovigilance in Canada is the duty of Health Canada. Adverse event reports are gathered and analysed using the Canada Vigilance database, pharmaceutical businesses are required to submit quarterly safety update reports to Health Canada.

f. World Health Organization (WHO): Through its global database of Individual Case Safety Reports (ICSRs), VigiBase, the World Health Organization (WHO) offers a global perspective on pharmacovigilance, it is a member of the WHO Collaborating Center for International Drug Monitoring and receives individual case safety reports from national pharmacovigilance centers throughout the world.

g. Other Countries: Several additional countries have established their own pharmacovigilance and safety databases, often based on international guidelines, in every country, pharmaceutical companies, clients, and medical professionals could have different reporting requirements, despite regional differences, efforts are being made globally to harmonize pharmacovigilance procedures and standards. Cooperation between regulatory agencies and adherence to international standards, including those set forth by the International Council for Harmonization of Technical Requirements for Pharmaceuticals for Human Use (ICH), promote a more standardized approach to drug safety monitoring on a global scale.

Regulatory Submissions: Reports that are expedited are sent to regulatory bodies via designated routes, frequently with the use of electronic technologies like the E2B format for individual case safety reports.

a. Signal Recognition:

Continuous Monitoring: Sponsors and regulatory agencies can notice possible safety issues or new patterns of unfavorable events with the aid of expedited reporting, which aids in continuous signal detection. Reports on Development Safety Updates (DSURs):

b. Aggregate Reporting: During the development phase, sponsors offer Development Safety Update Reports (DSURs), which summarize safety data and analysis, on a regular basis in addition to individual case reports.

c. Risk Control:

Risk minimizing: In order for regulatory bodies to properly protect the public's health, expedited reporting is essential to risk management and minimizing.

d. Interactions with Ethics Committees and Investigators:

Site Reporting: To guarantee that the proper steps are followed at the site level, investigators and ethical committees are frequently notified as soon as major and unexpected adverse occurrences occur.

e. After-Market Monitoring Sustaining Vigilance: During the post-marketing period, prompt reporting is crucial to tracking a product's actual safety profile, even after it has received regulatory approval, one essential element of pharmacovigilance is expedited reporting, which makes sure that new safety issues are found quickly and dealt with effectively to protect patients who are using medications, it encourages risk management to be proactive throughout a drug's lifecycle.

f. Safety reports for specific cases: Individual Case Safety Reports (ICSRs), which include comprehensive information regarding specific occurrences of adverse events or suspected adverse reactions connected to the use of a pharmaceutical product, are essential to pharmacovigilance. For evaluating the safety profile of medications and other medical items over the course of their lives, these reports are essential. The following are important details about safety reports for individual cases:

12.3. Individual case safety reports

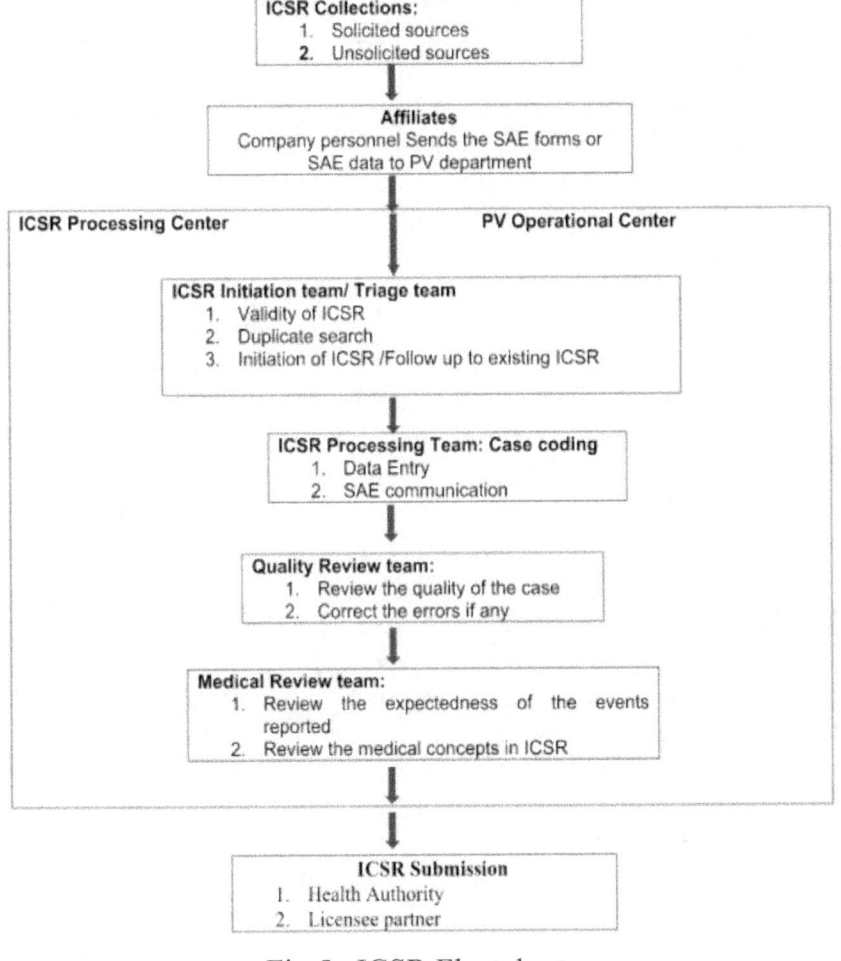

Fig.5. ICSR Flowchart

What is meant by ICSR?

An Individual Case Safety Report (ICSR) is a document that provides comprehensive details regarding a single untoward incident or possible unfavourable reaction associated with the administration of a pharmaceutical. Usually, it includes details on the patient, the suspected medication, the adverse event, and any pertinent medical history.

What makes up an ICSR:

Patient Data: Personal characteristics, health history, and additional pertinent data.

Unfavourable occurrence details: A thorough account of the unfavourable reaction or occurrence, encompassing its beginning, progressing, intensity, and conclusion.

Suspected Medicinal Product: Details regarding the medication, such as dosage, mode of administration, and start and stop dates, that are thought to be connected to the adverse event.

Reporter Information: Specifics about the individual or organization that filed the adverse event report.

Other Relevant Information: Extra details that could be important to comprehending the incident, such as concurrent drug use or pre-existing medical issues.

The ICSRs' source:

Healthcare Professionals: Those who watch and record adverse events in clinical practice are frequently the source of reports.

Patients: First-hand accounts from patients who encounter unfavourable outcomes.

Regulatory Authorities: Reports can be sent directly to regulatory agencies or via pharmacovigilance systems.

Sponsors: Pharmaceutical companies are in charge of gathering and submitting ICSRs as sponsors of clinical studies or holders of marketing authorization.

Fast Track Reporting:

Requirements for Accelerated Reporting: Regulatory authorities may need to receive reports of some adverse events—especially those that are serious and unexpected—in an expedited manner and within a certain amount of time.

timetables: Depending on the severity and circumstances of the adverse event, expedited reporting timetables can vary, but they often require reporting within 7 or 15 calendar days.

ICSR Data Uniformity:
ICH E2B Format: The ICH E2B format offers sponsors and regulatory bodies a uniform electronic framework for exchanging ICSRs. It makes data sharing easier and guarantees consistency.

Finding and Analyzing Signals:
Signal Detection: Aggregated ICSR analysis aids in the identification of possible safety signals or new trends that might point to hazards that were not previously known.
Data mining: To find patterns and correlations, sophisticated data mining techniques can be used on big databases of ICSRs.

Reporting in aggregate:
Development Safety Update Reports (DSURs): During the development phase, sponsors offer periodic aggregate safety reports, such DSURs, which synthesize safety data across certain time intervals. These reports are in addition to the individual reports.

Parts in the Management of Risk:
Risk Assessment: To guarantee the safe use of pharmaceuticals, ICSRs support continuing risk assessment and management initiatives.
Risk-Benefit Assessment: ICSRs are used by regulatory bodies to evaluate the overall risk-benefit ratio of a pharmaceutical product.
Interaction & Cooperation:

Communication with Healthcare Professionals: In order to update product labels or distribute safety information, ICSRs may initiate contact with healthcare professionals.
Cooperation with Regulatory Authorities: In order to exchange ICSRs and support pharmacovigilance initiatives, sponsors work with regulatory authorities in tandem.

After-Market Monitoring Ongoing Monitoring: To keep an eye on a product's actual safety profile in the real world, ICSRs are gathered and examined throughout the post-marketing stage, **Individual Case Safety Reports** are essential to pharmacovigilance initiatives because they support sponsors, regulatory bodies, and medical practitioners in tracking and addressing the safety of pharmaceuticals, thereby guaranteeing patient safety and public health in general.

12.4. Regular reports on safety updates: Periodic Safety Update Reports (PSURs)—also referred to as Periodic Benefit-Risk Evaluation Reports (PBRERs)—are thorough reports that marketing authorization holders (MAHs) provide to regulatory bodies at predetermined intervals throughout a medication's post-approval phase. PSURs offer a methodical and comprehensive summary of the safety profile of the product by combining information from multiple sources, such as scientific publications, post-marketing surveillance, and clinical trials. The following are important elements of periodic safety update reports:

Why PSURs are used:
Frequent Safety Monitoring: PSURs are used to methodically and frequently keep an eye on a drug's safety during the course of its post-approval lifecycle.
Benefit-Risk Assessment: Using the available safety data, the reports enable a thorough benefit-risk assessment.
Regularity of Submission:
Period: The frequency of PSUR submissions is specified by regulatory bodies; it is usually once a year for the first few years following approval and then less frequently after that.

PSUR contents:
a. Cumulative Safety Data: An extensive summary of safety information, including adverse drug responses, major adverse events, and adverse events reported globally.
b. Clinical Trial Data: An overview of completed and continuing clinical trials, together with information on safety.

c. Review of the Literature: An analysis of pertinent scientific research for information on safety.

d. Risk-Benefit Assessment: Evaluation of the product's overall risk-benefit profile.

e. Signal Detection and Analysis: This process involves locating and examining emerging safety concerns, trends, or signals.

f. Current Situation of Risk Management Measures: Reports on the efficiency and state of risk management initiatives.

g. Sources of Data for PSURs: Combined information from individual case reports, especially concerning and unanticipated adverse events, is found in Individual Case Safety Reports (ICSRs).

h. Clinical Trials: Combining results on safety from both finished and continuing clinical trials.

i. Post-Marketing Surveillance: Information gathered through systems of spontaneous reporting and post-marketing surveillance operations.

Minimizing and mitigating risks:
Risk Management Plan (RMP): PSURs may contain information on how well the risk reduction and minimization strategies described in the RMP are being implemented.

Worldwide Harmonization:
International Council for Harmonization of Technical Requirements for Pharmaceuticals for Human Use (ICH) Guidelines: PSURs are created in compliance with ICH E2C in particular.

Submission to the Authorities in Charge:
a. Regulatory Compliance: In accordance with national and international laws, PSURs must be filed to regulatory bodies.

b. Electronic Submission: Submissions are frequently made electronically, following the formats and instructions set forth by regulatory bodies.

Working together with regulatory bodies:
a. Communication: Regarding safety concerns found in PSURs, MAHs and regulatory agencies should continue to communicate and work together.

b. Follow-Up Measures: In light of the conclusions in PSURs, regulatory bodies may make requests for more information or suggest taking additional measures.

Function in Signal Recognition:
Early Signal Detection: PSURs are involved in the early identification of signals pertaining to possible safety issues.
Signal Analysis: Carefully examining safety data enables the identification of trends or patterns that could need more research.

Revision of Product Labelling:
Labelling Changes: In the event that new safety information or modifications to the benefit-risk profile are required, PSURs may result in product label adjustments.

Periodic Safety Update Reports help the continued assessment and management of the safety of pharmaceuticals during the post-marketing phase by supporting pharmacovigilance initiatives, these are crucial records that support the preservation of public health and guarantee the continued safe administration of medications.

12.5. Accelerated reporting following approval: Post-approval expedited reporting pertains to the prompt submission of safety data, namely adverse events or suspected adverse responses, to regulatory bodies following the issuance of a marketing license for a pharmaceutical product, a drug's safety profile must be continuously monitored even after it has been given the all-clear to be marketed in order to spot and resolve any new or developing safety issues, the following are important elements of rapid reporting upon approval:

Reporting Adverse Events: Any unfavourable medical incident connected to a patient's usage of a medication product is defined as an adverse event, this covers adverse reactions, prescription mistakes, problems with product quality, and any other unforeseen or unplanned incidents.

Reporting Requirement: In compliance with certain rules and standards, marketing authorization holders (MAHs) are usually obliged to report adverse incidents to regulatory authorities.

Unexpected and Serious Adverse Events:

Reporting Requirements: Serious and unforeseen adverse events, such as those that pose a threat to life, necessitate hospitalization, result in a chronic or major handicap or incapacity, or cause congenital abnormalities, are frequently the focus of post-approval expedited reporting.

Reporting Schedules:

Regulation Requirements: Post-approval expedited reporting deadlines differ depending on the regulatory body and the location. Depending on the seriousness and nature of the adverse event, reporting may be needed in 15 calendar days, 30 calendar days, or other time periods.

Standards and Guidance for Regulation:

ICH rules: Post-approval expedited reporting is governed by the International Council for Harmonization of Technical Requirements for Pharmaceuticals for Human Use (ICH) rules, specifically ICH E2D.

Local Regulation Requirements: MAHs are required to comply with the particular laws and mandates on reporting that are in place in the nations or areas in which their goods are approved.

Databases and Systems for Safety:

Maintenance of Safety Databases: To gather and handle post-approval safety data, MAHs keep up safety databases.

Electronic Reporting Systems: Standardized forms, such the ICH E2B format for Individual Case Safety Reports, are frequently used to submit expedited reports electronically.

Finding and Analysing Signals:

Continuous Monitoring: By assisting regulatory bodies and MAHs in identifying possible safety signals or new patterns of adverse

events, post-approval expedited reporting helps with continued signal detection.
Data Analysis: Post-approval safety data aggregated analysis aids in evaluating the product's overall safety profile.

Risk Control:
Risk Assessment: To guarantee the safe use of pharmaceuticals, post-approval rapid reporting facilitates continuing risk assessment and risk management initiatives.
Risk Minimization Measures: In light of the results of the post-approval safety reporting, MAHs may decide to take further steps to reduce risk.

Interaction with Regulatory Bodies:
Regulatory Interaction: To share post-approval safety results, offer updates, and answer any regulatory questions or concerns, MAHs keep constant lines of communication open with regulatory authorities.
Answers to Regulatory Requests: In the event that regulatory authorities ask for more information, MAHs are required to provide it as soon as possible.

International Cooperation: The international markets, MAHs work together with regulatory bodies throughout the globe to exchange safety data and support pharmacovigilance initiatives on a global scale.

Modifications to Product Labels:
Labelling Changes: Updates to product labels, such as modifications to warnings, precautions, or contraindications, may result from new safety information discovered through post-approval accelerated reporting, post-approval accelerated reporting is an essential part of pharmacovigilance after marketing. It helps to maintain patient safety and a positive benefit-risk profile for pharmaceuticals by making ensuring that any new safety issues pertaining to drugs that have been marketed are quickly found and reported to regulatory bodies.

12.6. Planning for pharmacovigilance:

Planning for pharmacovigilance entails methodically creating and putting into action plans and initiatives to keep an eye on and guarantee the security of pharmaceuticals at every stage of their lives. Pre-approval (clinical development) and post-approval phases are included, and its goal is to detect, evaluate, and control hazards related to the use of pharmaceuticals. Aspects that are crucial to pharmacovigilance planning include:

a. Overview of Pharmacovigilance Planning: Pharmacovigilance planning is a methodical and anticipatory technique to tracking and guaranteeing the security of pharmaceuticals.

b. Viewpoint on the Lifecycle: This covers organizing tasks from early clinical development to post-marketing monitoring.

c. Regulations and Recommendations:

Compliance: Planning needs to follow the rules and regulations set forth by health authorities (FDA, EMA, etc.).

d. ICH recommendations: Pharmacovigilance planning is aided by the International Council for Harmonization of Technical Requirements for Pharmaceuticals for Human Use (ICH) recommendations, which include ICH E2E.

Master File for the Pharmacovigilance System (PSMF):

Documentation: Businesses can keep a complete record of their pharmacovigilance system, including planning activities, in a Pharmacovigilance System Master File (PSMF).

Pharmacovigilance Planning Components:

The creation and application of risk management plans (RMPs), which include techniques for risk reduction and mitigation, techniques for identifying and controlling signals that could raise safety issues are referred to as signal detection and management.

Expedited Reporting: Post-approval expedited reporting is one of the processes for promptly informing regulatory bodies of adverse events.

Safety Communication: Strategies for informing patients, healthcare providers, and government agencies about safety information.

Clinical Development and Integration:
Early Planning: Including safety monitoring in clinical trials, pharmacovigilance issues are integrated into the early phases of drug development.

Processes and Informed Consent: Creating papers and processes pertaining to safety reporting and monitoring.

Education and Training:
Employee Education: Ensuring that pertinent staff members receive instruction on pharmacovigilance protocols and guidelines, ongoing training to keep employees informed about new advancements and legal needs is known as continuous education.

Gathering and Organizing Data:
Individual Case Safety Reports (ICSRs) and other safety data are collected and managed through the establishment and upkeep of safety databases, ensuring the precision and caliber of safety data gathered is known as data quality.

Inspections and Audits for Pharmacovigilance:
Conducting internal audits is one way to evaluate the pharmacovigilance system's compliance and efficacy.

Regulatory Inspections: Being ready for and handling pharmacovigilance-related regulatory inspections.

Global Pharmacovigilance Markets:
Working with regulatory bodies around the world and addressing pharmacovigilance requirements in different locations is known as international collaboration.

Harmonization: Ensuring uniformity by coordinating pharmacovigilance efforts with international standards.

Strategies for Surveillance After Approval:
Planning and submitting Periodic Safety Update Reports (PSURs) is the process of giving regulatory bodies thorough safety updates.

Signal Detection in Real-World Environments: Methods for keeping an eye out for safety signals in actual post-marketing environments.

Patient Assistance and Involvement: Patient education refers to the application of techniques to inform patients about the proper and safe administration of pharmaceuticals.
Patient Reporting Programs: assisting and motivating patients to report unfavourable occurrences.

Constant Enhancement: Quality Management Systems: Quality management systems are put into place to guarantee that pharmacovigilance procedures are continuously improved, establishing procedures for gathering input and insights from safety monitoring operations and reported bad incidents is known as the "feedback mechanisms", the dynamic process of pharmacovigilance planning necessitates constant assessment and adjustment in response to new safety concerns, shifting conditions, and changing legal requirements, it is essential to maintaining the security of pharmaceuticals and safeguarding patients' health.

12.7. Pharmacovigilance best practices for clinicians: In order to guarantee the safety of clinical trial participants and the correct and trustworthy gathering of safety data, pharmacovigilance adheres to Good Clinical Practice (GCP), which is based on ethical and scientific principles. Although GCP has historically been linked to the execution of clinical trials, it also includes post-marketing monitoring of a drug's safety profile. The following are important GCP factors for pharmacovigilance:

Principles of Ethics: Obtain informed consent from patients or research participants prior to gathering safety data.
Protection of Participants: It is imperative to put trial participants' rights, security, and welfare first.

Adherence to Regulations: Respect for Regulations: Adhere to the national and international laws, rules, and directives pertaining to pharmacovigilance procedures.
ICH recommendations: Adhere to GCP and pharmacovigilance-related International Council for Harmonization of Technical Requirements for Pharmaceuticals for Human Use (ICH) recommendations.

Monitoring and Reporting Safety:
Adverse Event Reporting: During clinical trials and post-marketing surveillance, establish methodical protocols for the gathering, evaluation, and reporting of adverse events.
Follow the deadlines for reporting major and unanticipated adverse events to regulatory bodies in an expeditious manner.

Protocol Creation:
Study protocols should incorporate safety monitoring techniques and include instructions on how to gather, report, and analyse safety data, create risk management plans, or RMPs, to oversee and lessen possible risks related to the investigational product.

Management of Safety Databases:
Data Integrity and Quality: Take steps to guarantee the integrity, accuracy, and quality of safety data that has been gathered and stored in databases.
Data Coding and Standardization: To enable uniform reporting, use established coding systems (such as MedDRA) for adverse events.

Education and Training:
Personnel Training: Make certain that all participants in pharmacovigilance operations have received sufficient instruction on GCP guidelines and the necessity of filing safety reports.
Ongoing Education: To keep staff members informed about modifications to laws and industry best practices, offer continuing education.

Record-keeping:
Study Documentation: Keep thorough and accurate records of all safety-related activities, including as safety updates, adverse event reports, and investigator brochures.
Documentation: Define protocols for the methodical and structured documentation of safety information.

Reports on Safety to Ethics Committees:
Notifications to Ethics Committees: Immediately notify ethics committees of any modifications to the investigational product's safety profile that may have an impact on the security of participants.

Finding and Analysing Signals:
Signal Detection Protocols: Put protocols in place for the methodical identification and evaluation of safety signals.
Risk-Benefit Analysis: Regularly analyse risks and benefits to determine how safe an investigational product is overall.

Audits and Inspections:
Being Ready for Audits: Be ready for both internal and external audits that are intended to evaluate your adherence to GCP and pharmacovigilance regulations.
Remedial Actions: Take remedial measures to address any shortcomings found during audits or inspections.

Interaction & Cooperation:
Communication Plans: Create communication plans for informing investigators, sponsors, authorities in charge of regulations, and other pertinent parties about safety matters.
Cooperation with Regulatory Authorities: When it comes to safety-related issues, cooperate and communicate openly with regulatory authorities.

Post-Marketing Monitoring, Sustained Vigilance: To guarantee continuous safety monitoring in actual environments, extend GCP principles to post-marketing surveillance.
Post-Approval Studies: If necessary, carry out post-approval investigations to evaluate the marketed product's safety in more detail, throughout a medical product's lifecycle, upholding the highest standards of safety and moral behaviour in pharmacovigilance requires adherence to GCP principles. It contributes to the general integrity of the drug development process, safeguards the rights of study participants and patients, and ensures the accuracy of safety data.

Unit 5

Chapter 13
Pharmacogenomics of adverse drug reactions

Pharmacogenomics refers to the study of how an individual's genetic makeup influences their response to drugs. Adverse Drug Reactions (ADRs) are unwanted and harmful effects associated with the use of medications. Understanding the pharmacogenomics of adverse drug reactions involves investigating how genetic variations can contribute to an individual's susceptibility to experiencing adverse effects or, in some cases, predict the likelihood of a favorable response to a drug.

Genetic Variation:
Polymorphisms: Genetic polymorphisms, variations in DNA sequences among individuals, can influence drug metabolism, transport, and target interactions.

Inherited Traits: Many of these polymorphisms are inherited and can impact an individual's ability to metabolize or respond to specific drugs.

Drug Metabolism Enzymes:
Cytochrome P450 (CYP) Enzymes: Genetic variations in CYP enzymes, responsible for drug metabolism in the liver, can affect the rate at which drugs are processed and eliminated.

Poor Metabolizers and Ultrarapid Metabolizers: Some individuals may be classified as poor metabolizers, leading to increased drug concentrations and a higher risk of adverse reactions, while ultrarapid metabolizers may experience reduced drug efficacy.

Drug Transporters:
ATP-Binding Cassette (ABC) Transporters: Genetic variations in drug transporters can impact the absorption, distribution, and elimination of drugs, influencing their efficacy and safety.

Multidrug Resistance Protein (MRP) and P-Glycoprotein (P-gp): Variations in these transporters can affect drug disposition and contribute to adverse effects.

HLA Genes and Immunogenetic Factors:

HLA-B and HLA-DRB1: Certain human leukocyte antigen (HLA) genes have been associated with hypersensitivity reactions to specific drugs, such as abacavir (HLA-B57:01) and allopurinol (HLA-B58:01).

Stevens-Johnson Syndrome (SJS) and Toxic Epidermal Necrolysis (TEN): Severe cutaneous adverse reactions, like SJS and TEN, have been linked to specific HLA alleles in response to certain drugs.

Clozapine and Agranulocytosis:

HLA-DQB1: Genetic variations in the HLA-DQB1 gene have been associated with an increased risk of clozapine-induced agranulocytosis in individuals with schizophrenia.

Warfarin Sensitivity:

VKORC1 and CYP2C9: Variations in the VKORC1 and CYP2C9 genes influence an individual's response to warfarin, a commonly used anticoagulant. Genetic testing helps in dose optimization to avoid bleeding or insufficient anticoagulation.

Abacavir Hypersensitivity:

HLA-B*57:01: Genetic testing for the presence of HLA-B*57:01 is recommended before prescribing abacavir to prevent hypersensitivity reactions in HIV patients.

Statins and Myopathy:

SLCO1B1: Polymorphisms in the SLCO1B1 gene have been linked to an increased risk of statin-induced myopathy.

Implementation of Pharmacogenomics:

Genetic Testing: The use of genetic testing to identify relevant genetic variants before drug prescription is becoming more common, especially for drugs with known pharmacogenomic associations.

Clinical Decision Support: Integration of pharmacogenomic information into clinical decision support systems to guide personalized prescribing.

Challenges and Future Directions:
Complexity: Pharmacogenomics is complex, and multiple genetic and environmental factors may contribute to adverse reactions.
Research and Discovery: Ongoing research aims to identify new pharmacogenomic associations and enhance our understanding of the genetic basis of adverse drug reactions.
Understanding the pharmacogenomics of adverse drug reactions holds great promise for personalized medicine, where drug therapy can be Targeted to an individual's genetic makeup to maximize efficacy and minimize the risk of adverse effects. Incorporating pharmacogenomic information into clinical practice has the potential to enhance drug safety and optimize therapeutic outcomes.

13.1. Genetics related ADR with example focusing PK parameters: Adverse drug reactions (ADRs) influenced by genetics, particularly those related to pharmacokinetic (PK) parameters, highlight how genetic variations can impact drug metabolism, absorption, distribution, and elimination. Here are examples of ADRs with a focus on PK parameters influenced by genetic factors:

Warfarin and CYP2C9/VKORC1 Variants:
PK Parameter Affected: Warfarin, an anticoagulant, undergoes metabolism primarily through the cytochrome P450 enzyme CYP2C9, additionally, VKORC1 is involved in the vitamin K cycle, influencing warfarin sensitivity.
Genetic Influence: Genetic variations in the CYP2C9 gene result in different metabolic rates for warfarin. Polymorphisms in VKORC1 can affect sensitivity to warfarin.
ADRs: Variability in drug response may lead to an increased risk of bleeding in individuals with reduced CYP2C9 activity or specific VKORC1 variants.

Codeine and CYP2D6 Polymorphism:

PK Parameter Affected: Codeine is metabolized to its active form, morphine, by the cytochrome P450 enzyme CYP2D6.

Genetic Influence: Individuals with different CYP2D6 genotypes metabolize codeine at varying rates. Poor metabolizers may experience reduced conversion to morphine, leading to decreased analgesic efficacy.

ADRs: Poor metabolizers may not achieve sufficient pain relief, while ultra-rapid metabolizers may be at risk of opioid toxicity.

Clopidogrel and CYP2C19 Polymorphism:

PK Parameter Affected: Clopidogrel is a prodrug activated by CYP2C19 to its active metabolite, which inhibits platelet aggregation.

Genetic Influence: Genetic variations in CYP2C19 affect the conversion of clopidogrel to its active form. Poor metabolizers have reduced efficacy.

ADRs: Poor metabolizers are at an increased risk of cardiovascular events due to diminished antiplatelet effects.

Tacrolimus and CYP3A5 Polymorphism:

PK Parameter Affected: Tacrolimus, an immunosuppressive drug, is metabolized by CYP3A enzymes.

Genetic Influence: CYP3A5 polymorphisms affect the metabolism of tacrolimus. Non-expressers of CYP3A5 may have higher drug concentrations.

ADRs: Non-expressers may be at risk of tacrolimus toxicity, while expressers may require higher doses to achieve therapeutic levels.

Isoniazid and NAT2 Polymorphism:

PK Parameter Affected: Isoniazid, used for tuberculosis treatment, is metabolized by N-acetyltransferase 2 (NAT2).

Genetic Influence: NAT2 polymorphisms result in slow, intermediate, or fast acetylator phenotypes, affecting isoniazid metabolism.

ADRs: Slow acetylators may experience higher isoniazid concentrations, leading to an increased risk of peripheral neuropathy.

Statins and SLCO1B1 Polymorphism:

PK Parameter Affected: Statins, such as simvastatin, undergo hepatic uptake by organic anion-transporting polypeptide 1B1 (OATP1B1), encoded by SLCO1B1.

Genetic Influence: Polymorphisms in SLCO1B1 can affect the hepatic uptake of statins.

ADRs: Reduced function variants may lead to increased statin concentrations, potentially increasing the risk of myopathy or rhabdomyolysis.

Chapter 14
Drug safety evaluation in special population

Understanding the pharmacogenomics of these examples helps tailor drug therapy to individual patients, optimizing efficacy while minimizing the risk of adverse effects. Incorporating genetic testing into clinical decision-making can enhance personalized medicine approaches for safer and more effective drug treatments.

14.1. Pediatrics in pharmacovigilance:

Pharmacovigilance in pediatrics involves the systematic monitoring and evaluation of the safety of medications in children. Children often differ from adults in terms of physiology, pharmacokinetics, and drug response, making it crucial to assess and manage potential risks associated with the use of pharmaceutical products in this population.

Dose Adjustments and Formulations:
Children may require age- and weight-appropriate dosing adjustments due to variations in drug metabolism and clearance.
Development of pediatric-friendly formulations, such as liquid formulations or chewable tablets, to facilitate accurate and safe administration.

Pharmacokinetic and Pharmacodynamic Variability:
Pediatric patients may exhibit variability in drug absorption, distribution, metabolism, and elimination, which can influence drug exposure, understanding the developmental changes in pharmacokinetics and pharmacodynamics across different age groups is crucial for appropriate dosing.

Off-Label Use and Unlicensed Medicines: Off-label use (use of a drug in a manner not approved by regulatory authorities) is common in pediatrics due to the limited number of medications specifically approved for children, monitoring and reporting adverse events associated with off-label and unlicensed drug use in pediatric patients.

Special Populations: Neonates and premature infants often have unique pharmacokinetic profiles and may require specialized attention in pharmacovigilance, monitoring drug safety in specific pediatric populations, such as those with chronic illnesses or genetic conditions, where drug response may vary.

Adverse Event Reporting: Ensuring timely and accurate reporting of adverse drug reactions (ADRs) in pediatric patients to regulatory authorities, encouraging healthcare providers, parents, and caregivers to report suspected adverse events associated with drug use in children.

Pediatric-Specific Regulatory Guidelines:
Regulatory agencies, such as the U.S. Food and Drug Administration (FDA) and the European Medicines Agency (EMA), provide specific guidelines for the development and monitoring of drugs in the pediatric population, compliance with pediatric regulatory requirements for conducting pediatric clinical trials and reporting safety data.

Pediatric Pharmacovigilance Research: Conducting research to assess the long-term safety and effectiveness of drugs used in pediatric populations, studying the impact of drug therapy on growth, development, and neurocognitive outcomes in children.

Communication and Education: Communicating safety information to healthcare professionals, parents, and caregivers to enhance awareness of potential risks, providing education on the importance of reporting adverse events in pediatric patients.

Collaboration and Data Sharing: Collaboration between healthcare providers, regulatory agencies, and pharmaceutical companies to share safety data and improve pediatric pharmacovigilance, participation in international initiatives to enhance the global understanding of pediatric drug safety.

Registry studies and real-world evidence: Establishing and utilizing pediatric drug registries to monitor the safety of medications in real-world settings, utilizing real-world evidence to complement data from clinical trials and provide insights into the safety of drugs used in routine pediatric care.

Pediatrics is a branch of medicine that focuses on the health and well-being of infants, children, and adolescents. This specialized field addresses the unique medical needs and considerations associated with different stages of childhood development. Here are key aspects of pediatrics:

Age Ranges:
Infants: Birth to 1 year
Toddlers: 1 to 3 years
Preschoolers: 3 to 6 years
School-age children: 6 to 12 years
Adolescents: 12 to 18 years

Pediatric Healthcare Providers:
a. Pediatricians: Medical doctors specializing in the care of children.
b. Pediatric Nurses: Nurses with expertise in caring for pediatric patients.
c. Pediatric Subspecialists: Healthcare professionals who focus on specific pediatric specialties (e.g., pediatric cardiologists, pediatric neurologists).

Growth and Development:
Milestones: Monitoring and assessing developmental milestones in areas such as motor skills, language, and socialization.
Immunizations: Administering vaccinations to protect against infectious diseases.

Common Pediatric Health Issues:
Respiratory Infections: Common cold, flu, bronchiolitis.
Gastrointestinal Disorders: Gastroenteritis, constipation, reflux.
Childhood Infections: Ear infections, strep throat, chickenpox.
Chronic Conditions: Asthma, diabetes, allergies.
Behavioral and Mental Health: Attention-deficit/hyperactivity disorder (ADHD), anxiety, depression.

Pediatric Preventive Care:
Well-Baby and Well-Child Visits: Regular check-ups to monitor growth, development, and address parental concerns.

Screenings: Vision and hearing screenings, developmental screenings.
Nutritional Guidance: Promoting healthy eating habits and addressing nutritional concerns.

Neonatology:
Neonatologists: Specialists in the care of newborns, especially those born prematurely or with medical conditions.
Neonatal Intensive Care Units (NICUs): Specialized units for the intensive care of newborns.

Pediatric Emergency Care:
Pediatric Emergency Departments: Equipped to handle emergencies involving children.
Pediatric Advanced Life Support (PALS): Specialized training for healthcare providers in pediatric emergency care.

Pediatric Pharmacology:
Dosage Adjustments: Suspected medication dosages based on weight and age.
Child-Friendly Formulations: Developing liquid or chewable formulations for ease of administration.

Child Advocacy:
Child Safety: Promoting safety measures, including car seat use, childproofing homes, and preventing accidents.
Immunization Advocacy: Encouraging and educating parents on the importance of vaccinations.

Pediatric Surgery:
Pediatric Surgeons: Specializing in surgical procedures for children.
Common Procedures: Appendectomy, hernia repair, congenital anomaly correction.

Childhood Obesity Prevention:
Nutritional Counseling: Addressing diet and exercise to prevent and manage childhood obesity.

Physical Activity Promotion: Encouraging regular physical activity for overall health.

Adolescent Medicine:
Teen Health: Addressing the unique health needs and concerns of adolescents.
Reproductive Health: Providing guidance on puberty, sexual health, and contraception.

Family-Centered Care:
Inclusive Approach: Involving parents and caregivers in the decision-making process and care of the child.
Communication: Open and effective communication with both children and their families.
Pediatrics is a dynamic and evolving field that requires a holistic approach, considering not only the physical health but also the emotional and social well-being of the child. Continuous research and advancements in pediatric medicine contribute to improving the health outcomes and quality of life for children worldwide, pharmacovigilance in pediatrics is critical for ensuring the ongoing safety of medications used in children and minimizing the risks associated with drug therapy. It requires a collaborative and multidisciplinary approach involving healthcare professionals, regulatory agencies, industry stakeholders, and parents or caregivers to create a comprehensive understanding of drug safety in pediatric populations.

Drug safety evaluation in Pediatrics: Drug safety evaluation in pediatrics is a critical aspect of ensuring the well-being of children receiving pharmaceutical treatments. Pediatric patients, due to their unique physiological and developmental characteristics, may respond differently to medications compared to adults.

Pediatric Clinical Trials:
Ethical Considerations: Conducting clinical trials in children requires special ethical considerations, including informed consent and assent, as well as involvement of parents or guardians.

Age Stratification: Designing clinical trials with age-appropriate stratifications to account for developmental differences across pediatric age groups.

Pharmacokinetics and Pharmacodynamics:
Age-Related Changes: Understanding how drug absorption, distribution, metabolism, and elimination change with age in pediatric patients.
Dose Adjustments: Implementing age- and weight-appropriate dosing to account for differences in drug clearance and metabolism.
Pediatric Pharmacogenomics:
Genetic Variability: Considering genetic factors that may influence drug metabolism and response in pediatric patients.
Individualized Treatment: Suspected drug therapy based on pharmacogenomic information to optimize efficacy and minimize adverse reactions.

Age-Appropriate Formulations:
Liquid Formulations: Developing age-appropriate formulations such as liquids, suspensions, or chewable tablets to facilitate accurate dosing in young children.
Palatability: Ensuring palatability to improve medication adherence in pediatric patients.

Off-Label Use:
Monitoring Off-Label Use: Recognizing that many drugs are used off-label in pediatrics due to limited approved options.
Safety Surveillance for Off-Label Use: Systematically monitoring and evaluating the safety of off-label drug use in pediatric populations.

Long-Term Safety and Follow-up:
Long-Term Effects: Assessing the potential long-term safety of medications, especially those used for chronic conditions.
Follow-up Studies: Conducting post-marketing surveillance and follow-up studies to monitor for delayed adverse effects.

Registry Studies:
Pediatric Registries: Establishing and utilizing pediatric drug registries to track safety outcomes in real-world clinical settings.
Observational Data: Using real-world data from registries to complement findings from clinical trials and provide a broader understanding of drug safety.

Adverse Event Reporting:
Reporting Systems: Encouraging healthcare professionals, parents, and caregivers to report any adverse events or unexpected reactions associated with pediatric drug use.
Timely Reporting: Ensuring prompt reporting of adverse events to regulatory authorities to facilitate quick safety assessments.

Communication and Education:
Healthcare Provider Communication: Facilitating communication between healthcare providers, parents, and caregivers about potential risks and benefits of medications.
Patient and Family Education: Providing clear and accessible information to parents and caregivers about medication use, potential side effects, and the importance of reporting adverse events.

Pediatric-Specific Risk Management Plans:
Risk-Benefit Assessment: Conducting thorough risk-benefit assessments for pediatric medications, considering the specific context of use.
Risk Management Strategies: Implementing risk management plans that address pediatric safety concerns, including labeling, education, and monitoring.

Collaboration with Regulatory Agencies:
Regulatory Oversight: Collaborating with regulatory agencies to adhere to pediatric-specific regulatory requirements.
Post-Marketing Commitments: Fulfilling post-marketing commitments related to pediatric safety assessments as stipulated by regulatory authorities.

Continuous Surveillance and Improvement:
Continuous Monitoring: Implementing continuous surveillance systems to monitor the safety of pediatric medications throughout their lifecycle.

Adaptive Strategies: Employing adaptive strategies based on emerging safety data to enhance patient safety.

Drug safety evaluation in pediatrics requires a comprehensive and multidisciplinary approach, involving healthcare professionals, researchers, regulatory agencies, and parents or caregivers. It aims to strike a balance between providing effective treatments for pediatric conditions and minimizing the potential risks associated with medication use in this vulnerable population.

14.2. Pregnancy and lactation: Pregnancy and lactation introduce unique considerations in the use of medications, as the physiological changes during these periods can impact drug metabolism, distribution, and excretion. Ensuring the safety of medications for both the mother and the developing fetus or breastfeeding infant is crucial. Here are key aspects related to pregnancy and lactation:

a. Pregnancy:
Physiological Changes: Pregnancy alters the physiology of various organ systems, including changes in blood volume, cardiac output, and hormone levels, drug absorption, distribution, metabolism, and elimination may be affected during pregnancy.

Teratogenicity and Fetal Safety:
Teratogenicity: The potential to cause malformations in the developing fetus.

Teratogenic Classification: Drugs are categorized based on their potential fetal risk (e.g., FDA Pregnancy Categories, which include A, B, C, D, and X categories).

Fetal Development Stages: Drugs may have different effects at various stages of fetal development: The first trimester is particularly critical for organogenesis, and exposure during this time may pose a higher risk of congenital anomalies.

Risk-Benefit Assessment:
Balancing Risks and Benefits: Healthcare providers carefully assess the risks and benefits of medication use during pregnancy.
The severity of the maternal condition and the availability of alternative treatments are considered in the decision-making process.

Prenatal Screening and Monitoring:
Ultrasound and Monitoring: Prenatal screening, ultrasounds, and other monitoring tools help assess fetal development and detect any potential anomalies.

Common Medications During Pregnancy: Certain medications are considered generally safe during pregnancy, including some antibiotics, certain pain relievers (e.g., acetaminophen), and specific prenatal vitamins.

Avoidance of High-Risk Medications: Medications with known teratogenic effects or insufficient safety data may be avoided during pregnancy whenever possible.

Pregnancy Registries: Participation in pregnancy registries helps collect information on the safety of medications during pregnancy, these registries aid in monitoring outcomes and updating safety information.

b. Lactation:
Drug Transfer into Breast Milk:
Breast Milk Composition: The composition of breast milk and its potential to carry drugs into the infant's system.
Lipophilic vs. Hydrophilic Drugs: Lipophilic drugs are more likely to pass into breast milk.

Drug Safety during Breastfeeding:
Safety Considerations: Assessing the safety of medications during breastfeeding, considering potential effects on the infant.
Medications with Minimal Transfer: Identifying medications with minimal transfer into breast milk whenever possible.

Breastfeeding and Maternal Medication Use:
Timing of Medication Administration: Timing medication administration to minimize exposure during peak breastfeeding times.
Short Half-Life Drugs: Choosing medications with a short half-life when possible.

Common Medications during Lactation: Certain medications, such as some antibiotics, pain relievers (e.g., acetaminophen, ibuprofen), and specific antidepressants, are often considered compatible with breastfeeding.

Monitoring for Adverse Effects: Monitoring infants for potential adverse effects when mothers are taking medications during lactation, being aware of signs such as changes in feeding patterns, irritability, or changes in sleep.

Communication with Healthcare Providers:
Open communication between healthcare providers and breastfeeding mothers about medication use, seeking guidance from healthcare professionals to make informed decisions regarding medication safety during lactation.

Patient Education: Educating breastfeeding mothers about the safety of medications, potential risks, and the importance of consulting healthcare providers for personalized guidance, in both pregnancy and lactation, the safety of medications should be assessed on an individual basis. Healthcare providers play a crucial role in guiding pregnant and lactating individuals in making informed decisions regarding medication use, considering the specific circumstances of each patient. The goal is to optimize maternal health while minimizing potential risks to the developing fetus or breastfeeding infant.

Pregnancy and lactation in pharmacovigilance:
Pharmacovigilance in the context of pregnancy and lactation involves the systematic monitoring, detection, assessment, understanding, and prevention of adverse effects or any other drug-related problems during these critical periods. Ensuring the safety of medications for pregnant and lactating individuals is of utmost importance, as the physiological changes during these phases can impact drug metabolism and potential risks to the developing fetus or breastfeeding infant.

Pregnancy:
Adverse Event Reporting: Prompt reporting of adverse drug reactions (ADRs) observed during pregnancy to regulatory authorities, encouraging healthcare professionals and patients to report any suspected adverse events related to medication use during pregnancy.
Monitoring for Teratogenicity: Systematic monitoring for potential teratogenic effects of drugs, particularly during the critical periods of fetal development, assessing the safety of drugs used during pregnancy through epidemiological studies, registries, and clinical trials.

Pregnancy Registries: Utilizing pregnancy registries to collect and analyze data on the safety of medications used during pregnancy, collaborating with healthcare providers and pregnant individuals to contribute to pregnancy registry data.

Risk-Benefit Assessment:
Conducting comprehensive risk-benefit assessments for medications used during pregnancy, evaluating the severity of the maternal condition and the potential risks to the fetus against the benefits of treatment.

Labeling and Communication: Updating drug labels with relevant information on the safety profile during pregnancy, effective communication of risks and benefits to healthcare providers, pregnant individuals, and regulatory agencies.

International Collaboration: Collaborating internationally to share data and experiences related to the safety of medications during pregnancy, harmonizing pharmacovigilance efforts to improve the understanding of global trends and outcomes.

Lactation:
Breastfeeding and Adverse Event Reporting:
Vigilant monitoring and reporting of adverse events associated with medications used during lactation, encouraging healthcare providers and breastfeeding individuals to report any observed adverse effects in infants.

Drug Transfer into Breast Milk: Assessing the transfer of drugs into breast milk and monitoring for potential adverse effects in breastfeeding infants, studying pharmacokinetics to understand drug concentrations in breast milk.

Lactation Registries: Establishing lactation registries to gather data on the safety of medications during breastfeeding.
Collaborating with breastfeeding individuals and healthcare providers to contribute data to lactation registries.

Patient Education: Providing education to breastfeeding individuals about the safety of medications during lactation.
Promoting awareness of the importance of reporting any observed adverse effects in breastfeeding infants.
Communication with Healthcare Providers: Facilitating open communication between healthcare providers and breastfeeding individuals about medication use, offering guidance on the choice of medications compatible with breastfeeding.

Labeling and Information Dissemination: Ensuring drug labels include relevant information about the safety of medications during lactation, disseminating information to healthcare professionals and the public about the safety considerations of medications while breastfeeding.

Post-Marketing Surveillance: Continued post-marketing surveillance to identify and assess any potential safety concerns related to medications used during lactation, updating safety information based on emerging data and evidence, pharmacovigilance in pregnancy and lactation involves a comprehensive and ongoing effort to monitor, evaluate, and communicate the safety of medications, collaborative initiatives between regulatory agencies, healthcare providers, patients, and the pharmaceutical industry contribute to the collective understanding of drug safety during these critical periods. Regular updates to safety information and communication strategies enhance the overall pharmacovigilance process.

Drug safety evaluation in Pregnancy and lactation:
Drug safety evaluation in pregnancy and lactation is a critical aspect of ensuring the well-being of both the mother and the developing fetus or breastfeeding infant. The physiological changes that occur during these periods can impact drug metabolism, distribution, and excretion, necessitating a thorough assessment of the risks and benefits associated with medication use.

a. Pregnancy:
Risk Classification:
Teratogenicity Assessment: Evaluating the potential teratogenic effects of drugs, considering the risk of causing malformations in the developing fetus.
FDA Pregnancy Categories: Categorizing drugs based on potential fetal risk (e.g., Category A, B, C, D, X).

Pharmacokinetic Changes:
Physiological Changes: Recognizing physiological changes during pregnancy that may affect drug absorption, distribution, metabolism, and elimination.
Dose Adjustment: Adjusting drug dosages based on changes in drug pharmacokinetics to maintain therapeutic efficacy while minimizing risks.

Embryo-Fetal Developmental Studies:
Preclinical Studies: Conducting animal studies to assess the potential impact of drugs on embryo-fetal development.
Clinical Trials: Designing and conducting clinical trials with pregnant women to gather data on the safety profile of medications.

Registry Studies:
Pregnancy Registries: Establishing and utilizing pregnancy registries to monitor outcomes in pregnant women exposed to specific drugs.
Observational Data: Collecting observational data to assess the safety of medications used during pregnancy in real-world settings.

Risk-Benefit Assessment:
Individualized Assessment: Conducting a personalized risk-benefit assessment for each pregnant individual, considering the severity of the maternal condition and available treatment alternatives.
Shared Decision-Making: Involving healthcare providers and pregnant individuals in shared decision-making regarding medication use.

Communication and Education:
Healthcare Provider Communication: Ensuring open communication between healthcare providers and pregnant individuals about the potential risks and benefits of medications.
Patient Education: Providing information to pregnant individuals about the importance of medication adherence and reporting any adverse effects.

b. Lactation:
Drug Transfer into Breast Milk:
Breast Milk Composition: Understanding the composition of breast milk and the potential transfer of drugs into breast milk.
Lipophilic vs. Hydrophilic Drugs: Considering the characteristics of drugs that may affect their transfer into breast milk.

Pharmacokinetic Changes:
Postpartum Changes: Recognizing changes in drug metabolism and elimination during the postpartum period.

Dose Adjustment: Adjusting drug dosages to minimize infant exposure while maintaining therapeutic efficacy.

Risk-Benefit Assessment:
Assessing Infant Risk: Evaluating the potential risks to breastfeeding infants and balancing them against the benefits of maternal medication use.
Compatible Medications: Identifying medications that are considered compatible with breastfeeding.

Communication and Education:
Healthcare Provider Communication: Facilitating communication between healthcare providers and breastfeeding individuals about medication use during lactation.
Patient Education: Providing information to breastfeeding individuals about the safety considerations of medications and encouraging reporting of adverse effects in infants.

Breastfeeding Registries:
Establishment and Utilization: Creating breastfeeding registries to collect data on the safety of medications during lactation.
Observational Data: Gathering real-world data to assess the safety of medications used by breastfeeding individuals.

Labeling and Information Dissemination:
Inclusion of Safety Information: Ensuring that drug labels include relevant information regarding safety during lactation.
Disseminating Information: Disseminating information to healthcare professionals and the public about the safety of medications during breastfeeding.

Post-Marketing Surveillance:
Continuous Monitoring: Implementing continuous monitoring and surveillance to identify and assess any potential safety concerns related to medications used during lactation.

Updating Safety Information: Updating safety information based on emerging data and evidence, ensuring the safety of medications during pregnancy and lactation involves a comprehensive approach, including preclinical and clinical studies, real-world data collection, risk-benefit assessments, and effective communication with healthcare providers and individuals, the goal is to optimize maternal health outcomes while minimizing potential risks to the developing fetus or breastfeeding infant.

14.3. Geriatrics

Drug safety assessment in geriatrics is crucial due to the unique characteristics of the elderly population, including changes in physiology, pharmacokinetics, and pharmacodynamics. The following considerations should be made when assessing the safety of medications for the elderly:

i. Physiological Changes: People's bodies and the functions of their organs change with age, reduced lean body mass, increased body fat, and changes in liver and renal function can all affect drug distribution, metabolism, and excretion, the pharmacokinetics of drugs in elderly adults may change, necessitating dosage adjustments.

ii. Pharmacokinetics: Aging-related changes in medication absorption, distribution, metabolism, and elimination might affect a drug's pharmacokinetic profile, for example, decreased renal function may result in a slower excretion of medications, potentially leading to drug accumulation and toxicity.

iii. Polypharmacy: Older adults often take multiple medications to address various health conditions. Polypharmacy increases the risk of drug interactions, adverse effects, and non-adherence. Healthcare providers must be well knowledgeable about the potential interactions and cumulative effects of medications taken by elderly patients.

iv. Comorbidities: A large number of older people have many chronic conditions that may require taking multiple medications. The safety, effectiveness, and tolerance of drugs may be impacted by comorbidities. Clinicians should consider the patient's overall health before recommending medication.

v. Cognitive and Functional Impairment: Older adults may experience deterioration in their cognitive abilities and functional limitations. These factors might make it harder for patients to understand and adhere to prescribed regimens, which could have negative consequences. Medical practitioners should assess cognitive function and adjust drug regimens accordingly.

vi. Beers Criteria: The Beers Criteria for Potentially Inappropriate Medication Use in Older Adults is a technique that helps uncover medications that may pose increased hazards for older adults. Medical professionals need to be aware of these needs and take them into consideration when writing medications for elderly patients.

vii. Regular Monitoring: It's important to closely monitor the medication schedules of senior citizens. Frequent monitoring of organ function through laboratory tests and assessments of drug efficacy and potential adverse effects can help identify issues early and take necessary action.

viii. Patient education: It is crucial to provide senior patients with understandable information about the medications they take, including details on potential side effects, recommended dosages, and the importance of adhering to prescription schedules. This can increase patient involvement and reduce the likelihood of negative consequences.

ix. Customized Treatment Plans: It's critical to give each patient geriatric treatment that is unique to them, considering their goals, preferences, and state of health. Tailoring treatment options to the individual needs of older adults can optimize medication safety and overall healthcare outcomes.

x. Collaborative Healthcare Team: When delivering geriatric care, collaboration between physicians, pharmacists, nurses, and other professionals is essential. This multidisciplinary approach ensures that drug safety is thoroughly assessed and managed.

Chapter 15
CIOMS

Established internationally in 1949, the Council for International Organizations of Medical Sciences, sometimes known as CIOMS, is a non-governmental organization. Its purpose is to enhance public health by delivering advise on health research, specifically how to conduct human subjects' research ethically.

Among CIOMS's notable achievements is the development of ethical guidelines and best practices for the administration of biomedical research. The most well-known of these rules is the "CIOMS International Ethical Guidelines for Biomedical Research Involving Human Subjects". These guidelines offer a basis for moral considerations in the planning, carrying out, and disclosing of research involving human participants.

Among the main characteristics of the CIOMS guidelines are:
The phrase "informed consent" highlights the need of obtaining research participants' informed assent. It explains the principles of informed consent and why continuous communication is essential to the study.

Beneficence and Justice: Stresses the principles of beneficence (maximizing benefits and minimizing harm) and justice (fair distribution of the benefits and burdens of research). It is advised that researchers ensure equitable involvement and balance the benefits and drawbacks of their work.

The importance of social and scientific ideals in research is emphasized in the statement "Science and Social Value." Research projects should be designed to increase society's understanding, and their potential benefits should outweigh their drawbacks.

Vulnerable Populations: Provides specific guidance on how to incorporate susceptible populations, such as children, expecting women, and individuals with cognitive impairments. It is recommended that some groups be given more protection in order to ensure their welfare and rights.

Data and Safety Monitoring: It is advised that methods for tracking data and safety be put in place in order to supervise study progress and safeguard participants, promotes collaboration between the research communities and the investigators to ensure cultural sensitivity and honors local traditions and beliefs.

In addition, CIOMS collaborates with the World Health Organization (WHO) and other international organizations to promote ethical standards in global health research. For scientists doing biomedical research worldwide, ethics committees, and legislators, the CIOMS standards are a priceless resource.

The CIOMS principles are widely acknowledged and often included in institutional and national research ethics policies, but they are not required by law. Researchers and organizations worldwide refer to the CIOMS standards for guidance on ethical conduct in biomedical research involving human subjects.

15.1. CIOMS Working Groups: As of most current information update in January 2022, the Council for International Organizations of Medical Sciences, or CIOMS, contains a number of working committees that focus on specific aspects of medical sciences, research, and ethics. These working groups are intended to address specific problems, provide guidance, and support the advancement of international standards for medical research. Please be advised that the specific working groups and their topics of interest are subject to change at any time, the CIOMS working groups listed below are some examples as of my most current update:

Working Group on Vaccine Safety: Among other things related to vaccine safety, this group keeps an eye on and assesses adverse occurrences that follow vaccination. It could provide recommendations and guidelines to ensure the safe preparation and delivery of vaccines.

Working Group on Drug Safety: This group may address issues related to the safety of prescription drugs. It may address topics like pharmacovigilance, risk management, and evaluating the safety of drugs in a range of demographics.

For its advice on moral concerns in biomedical research involving human subjects, the CIOMS Working Group on Ethics in Medical Research is well known. The ethics working group may revise and develop these criteria to address emerging ethical concerns in medical research.

The primary focus of the Working Group on Standardized MedDRA Queries (SMQs) may be the development and maintenance of standardized MedDRA Queries, which are tools used by the regulatory and medical sectors for the standardized retrieval of specific safety information from the database.

Working Group on Pregnancy and Medication Creation: This group may address issues related to assessing the safety of medications during pregnancy, allowing pregnant mothers to take part in clinical trials, and the ethical dilemmas associated with developing medications for this population.

Working Group on Safe Medication delivery and Patient Involvement: Given the growing emphasis on patient-centered healthcare, this group may examine ways to involve patients in the formulation, evaluation, and safe delivery of pharmaceuticals.

It's important to confirm the most recent details regarding CIOMS's working groups by visiting their official website or contacting them directly, as organizational structures and goals are subject to change.

15.2. CIOMS Form:

SUSPECT ADVERSE REACTION REPORT

I. REACTION INFORMATION

1. PATIENT INITIALS (first, last)	1a. COUNTRY	2. DATE OF BIRTH			2a. AGE Years	3. SEX	4-6 REACTION ONSET			8-12 CHECK ALL APPROPRIATE TO ADVERSE REACTION
		Day	Month	Year			Day	Month	Year	

7 + 13 DESCRIBE REACTION(S) (including relevant tests/lab data)	8-12 CHECK ALL APPROPRIATE TO ADVERSE REACTION
	◌ PATIENT DIED
	◌ INVOLVED OR PROLONGED INPATIENT HOSPITALISATION
	◌ INVOLVED PERSISTENCE OR SIGNIFICANT DISABILITY OR INCAPACITY
	◌ LIFE THREATENING

II. SUSPECT DRUG(S) INFORMATION

14. SUSPECT DRUG(S) (include generic name)		20. DID REACTION ABATE AFTER STOPPING DRUG? ☐ YES ☐ NO ☐ NA
15. DAILY DOSE(S)	16. ROUTE(S) OF ADMINISTRATION	21. DID REACTION REAPPEAR AFTER REINTRODUCTION? ☐ YES ☐ NO ☐ NA
17. INDICATION(S) FOR USE		
18. THERAPY DATES (from/to)	19. THERAPY DURATION	

III. CONCOMITANT DRUG(S) AND HISTORY

22. CONCOMITANT DRUG(S) AND DATES OF ADMINISTRATION (exclude those used to treat reaction)
23. OTHER RELEVANT HISTORY (e.g. diagnostics, allergies, pregnancy with last month of period, etc.)

IV. MANUFACTURER INFORMATION

24a. NAME AND ADDRESS OF MANUFACTURER	
	24b. MFR CONTROL NO.
24c. DATE RECEIVED BY MANUFACTURER	24d. REPORT SOURCE ☐ STUDY ☐ LITERATURE ☐ HEALTH PROFESSIONAL
DATE OF THIS REPORT	25a. REPORT TYPE ☐ INITIAL ☐ FOLLOWUP

In the field of pharmacovigilance, the CIOMS (Council for International Organizations of Medical Sciences) Form is a form utilized for the recording of individual case safety reports (ICSRs). Pharmacovigilance refers to the study and methods of the detection, assessment, understanding, and prevention of adverse drug reactions or any other medication-related problems.

In collaboration with the International Conference on Harmonization of Technical Requirements for Registration of Pharmaceuticals for Human Use (ICH), CIOMS created a standard form for reporting adverse medication reactions. This form is known as the CIOMS I Report or CIOMS I Form.

Important features of the CIOMS I Form include:
Patient Information: Among other details, this section includes the patient's age, sex, weight, and relevant medical history.

Medication Information: Specifics about the suspected medication, including name, dosage, frequency, and duration of use

Adverse Event(s): A thorough description of the adverse event(s) or reaction(s), including the date they started, the extent of their severity, the outcome, and any actions they took in connection with the medicine.

Reporter Information: Name, address, and phone number of the individual who reported the negative incident.

Reaction(s) and Events(s): A full narrative of the adverse reaction or event, including applicable medical history and concomitant medicines.

Lab Data: Any important lab data relating to the unfortunate incidence.

Results: Information about the negative event's outcome, such as whether it resulted in a birth defect, hospitalization, disability, or other serious repercussions.

Drug(s) Exposure: Information on the patient's potential drug exposure, such as history of exposure and relapses.

Product Information: Details on the composition of the medication, including lot number and expiration date

Signature: The adverse event report's signer may have their own space on the form.

It's important to keep in mind that other standards and reporting systems are often utilized in pharmacovigilance in addition to the CIOMS I Form. The goal is to compile comprehensive, consistent data on adverse drug responses to support the assessment of the medication's safety profile.

It is not necessary to use the CIOMS I Form, but it does provide a methodical way to collect and report adverse drug reaction data, which aids in the global effort to ensure the safety of pharmaceutical products. Reporting requirements may vary between countries and regulatory agencies.

Chapter 16
CDSCO (India) and Pharmacovigilance

The Central Drugs Standard Control Organization (CDSCO) is the national regulatory organization in India that is in charge of medications and medical devices. CDSCO is crucial for ensuring the efficacy, safety, and quality of pharmaceuticals and medical equipment sold in India. As part of regulatory procedures, pharmacovigilance is also under the control of CDSCO.

Key components of CDSCO's pharmacovigilance efforts in India include the following:

1. India's Pharmacovigilance Program: The nation's pharmacovigilance efforts are overseen by the CDSCO. The Pharmacovigilance Program of India (PvPI) was established in 2010 with the intention of monitoring and compiling information on adverse drug reactions (ADRs) related to pharmaceutical products.

2. PvPI and ADR Monitoring: The CDSCO oversees the PvPI, which serves as the country's central location for ADR monitoring. It collaborates with several regional and national outlying centers, adverse drug reactions (ADRs) can be reported to the PvPI by pharmaceutical firms, consumers, and healthcare professionals via the ADR reporting form, mobile application, or website.

3. ADR Database: Using PvPI, CDSCO maintains a national ADR database that compiles, analyzes, and translates data regarding adverse reactions. This information is useful for both assessing the safety profiles of drugs and making regulatory decisions.

Two of CDSCO's duties include signal detection and risk management. They are executed by PvPI. Finding any safety concerns through data analysis is the technique of signal detection. By applying risk management strategies, hazards that have been identified can be minimized.

a. Training and Capacity Building: CDSCO and PvPI work together to provide training programs and workshops aimed at enhancing healthcare professionals' knowledge and proficiency in pharmacovigilance practices. Building capacity is necessary to ensure a robust pharmacovigilance system and improve the reporting culture.

b. International Cooperation: CDSCO collaborates with international organizations and regulatory bodies to enhance pharmacovigilance programs. Implementing industry best practices for pharmaceutical safety, participating in worldwide campaigns, and exchanging safety data are all part of this partnership.

c. Regulatory Oversight: CDSCO provides regulatory oversight to ensure that pharmaceutical companies follow pharmacovigilance laws. Submitting periodic safety update reports (PSURs) and other relevant safety information is part of this for marketing permission holders.

Tracking the safety of drugs over the duration of their lives is crucial, and CDSCO's involvement in pharmacovigilance demonstrates their commitment to protecting public health in India. The work of CDSCO supports continuous evaluations and improvements to the safety profiles of drugs supplied in India through PvPI.

16.1. D&C Act and Schedule Y:
Schedule Y and the Drugs and Cosmetics Act, 1940 are the main pieces of law in India that regulate the manufacture, import, distribution, and sale of pharmaceuticals and cosmetics. Below is a summary of the Drugs and Cosmetics Act and Schedule Y:

a. The Drugs and Cosmetics Act of 1940:
The Pharmaceuticals and Cosmetics Act, which was passed to ensure the efficacy, safety, and quality of the country's pharmaceutical and cosmetic products, is a comprehensive piece of legislation that regulates many aspects of the pharmaceutical and cosmetic industries in India, regulations can be established by the Central Government to guarantee that the Act's provisions are correctly implemented.

b. Schedule Y:

Schedule Y of the Drugs and Cosmetics Rules, 1945 discusses performing clinical trials for pharmaceutical items in India in specifically, it outlines the guidelines and requirements that sponsors, researchers, ethics committees, and other stakeholders involved in clinical trials need to follow, schedule Y provides a comprehensive description of the legal requirements and ethical concerns surrounding the conduct of clinical trials.

Crucial Information about Schedule Y:

Approval Process: The Controller General of Pharmaceuticals of India (DCGI) must grant approval prior to the start of clinical trials for new pharmaceuticals or investigational innovative medications (INDs). Schedule Y contains details about this.

Ethics Committee Approval: The schedule emphasizes that in order to ensure the safety and well-being of trial participants, it is the duty of the Ethics Committees to evaluate and approve clinical trial protocols.

Informed consent: This paper outlines the requirements that must be satisfied, together with the format and contents of the consent form, in order to obtain participants' informed consent, the obligations of sponsors and investigators for the tracking of clinical trials, the reporting of adverse events, and the timely submission of updates to regulatory agencies are outlined in Schedule Y.

Clinical Trial Registry: The schedule mandates that clinical trials be registered in a national clinical trial registry in order to increase openness.

Updates and Adjustments: Schedule Y has been modified in order to align it with the most recent international guidelines and clinical research best practices, over time, numerous changes have been made to improve participant safety, strengthen the regulatory framework, and speed up the approval processes for clinical studies, it's critical to keep in mind that Schedule Y must be followed by anyone planning or carrying out clinical studies in India. The schedule provides a framework to ensure that clinical trials are conducted ethically, considering the rights, safety, and well-being of trial participants. Investigators, sponsors, and regulatory agencies refer to Schedule Y as a guide for conducting clinical trials in India.

Schedule Y and the accompanying rules of the Medicines and Cosmetics Act, 1940, provide the legal framework for pharmaceuticals and cosmetics in India. An extensive synopsis of Schedule Y and the Drugs and Cosmetics Act can be found below:

a. The 1940 Drugs and Cosmetics Act's goals were:

The main goals of the Drugs and Cosmetics Act are to regulate the import, production, distribution, and retail sales of pharmaceuticals and cosmetics in order to guarantee their efficacy, safety, and quality. The Act gives the Central Government the authority to create regulations and appoint officials in order to achieve its objectives.

According to the Act, "drug" and "cosmetic" refer to both chemicals used in the diagnosis, treatment, mitigation, or prevention of illnesses as well as goods meant to be applied externally to the body for hygienic or cosmetic purposes.

Licenses and Permissions: The Act requires licenses to be obtained in order to distribute and manufacture cosmetics and pharmaceuticals. Only if certain conditions are achieved, like adherence to good manufacturing procedures (GMP), are licenses awarded.

Limitations and Guidelines: The Act states that owing to possible health risks, specific medications and cosmetics may be subject to limitations or outright bans.

Misbranding and Adulteration: Preventive measures are implemented to avoid mislabeled or altered medications and cosmetics. These include the need for appropriate packaging, precise labeling, and the ban on making exaggerated promises.

Examining Authorities and Examiners: Drug inspectors are empowered by the Act to look into locations, test substances, and take appropriate action when there is non-compliance.

Penalties and Offenses: The Act lists all violations and their associated punishments, including fines and jail time.

Schedule Y: The Drugs and Cosmetics Rules, 1945 regulate new drug approvals and clinical studies in particular. It has undergone modifications over time to guarantee the moral conduct of clinical research in India and to align it with global norms.

Important Details regarding Schedule Y: Approval procedure before starting clinical trials for new pharmaceuticals or investigational novel medicines (INDs), sponsors must obtain approval from the medicines Controller General of India (DCGI), complete information about the medication, its safety, and the trial protocol must be submitted as part of the application procedure.

Committee for Approval of Ethics: Schedule Y shows the role that Ethics Committees play in assessing and approving clinical trial techniques. The committees make sure that participant rights and safety are given first consideration and that the experiment is carried out ethically.

Consent that is informed: Comprehensive instructions are given for gaining participants' informed consent, including information on what should be included and how to format the consent form.

Observation and Documentation:
Schedule Y: Registry for Clinical Studies outlines the duties that sponsors and investigators have with regard to monitoring the progress of clinical studies, disclosing adverse events, and updating regulatory bodies on a regular basis, to improve openness, the timetable requires all clinical research to be reported in a national clinical trial registry.

After-Market Monitoring: It describes the procedures for post-marketing surveillance, which is necessary to keep an eye on the effectiveness and safety of medications once they are put on the market.

Modifications and Updates: The most recent worldwide standards and industry best practices for clinical research have been incorporated into Schedule Y, the modifications are intended to fortify the legal foundation and expedite the clinical trial approval procedure, investigators, sponsors, and regulatory agencies refer to Schedule Y as a manual for conducting clinical trials in India that guarantee compliance with legal and ethical standards. In order to get clearances and carry out clinical research in a way that puts participant safety and scientific integrity first, Schedule Y compliance is crucial.

16.2. Differences in Indian and global pharmacovigilance requirements:

Pharmacovigilance regulations are designed to ensure the safety of medicines by monitoring and assessing adverse drug reactions (ADRs) and putting the right safety measures in place to lower risks. Despite the fact that pharmacovigilance is governed by numerous international standards, various countries may have unique laws and customs. India and other countries have different standards for pharmacovigilance in the following significant ways:

1. International Standards Regulatory Organizations: Guidelines for international pharmacovigilance are provided by regulatory bodies such as the European Medicines Agency (EMA) and the U.S. Food and Drug Administration (FDA), as well as organizations such as the World Health Organization (WHO) and the International Council for Harmonization of Technical Requirements for Pharmaceuticals for Human Use (ICH).

Indian Measures: The Central Drugs Standard Control Organization (CDSCO) and the Pharmacovigilance Program of India (PvPI) oversee pharmacovigilance initiatives in India. The regulatory framework may have some unique quirks, but overall it complies with international norms.

2. Notifying the Unfavorable Event:

Global Conditions: Guidelines from around the world, such as those provided by the ICH, provide guidance on how to report adverse events that transpire in post-marketing surveillance and clinical studies.

Indian Measures: The National Coordination Centre for PvPI and the Pharmacovigilance Guidance Document are in charge of adverse event reporting in India. Certain forms and schedules that are unique to the Indian system may be followed by the reporting systems.

3. Worldwide specifications for the PSMF (Pharmacovigilance System Master File): The PSMF is a requirement for marketing authorization holders (MAHs) in the EU as evidence of the efficacy and adequacy of their pharmacovigilance systems.

Indian Measures: In compliance with PvPI standards, MAHs are expected to have robust pharmacovigilance mechanisms in place, even though a PSMF is not officially required in India.

4. Global Needs for Signal Management and Detection: Safety signal identification, assessment, and prioritization are governed by international standards as part of the signal detection and management process.

Indian Measures: The PvPI in India actively participates in signal identification and management, adhering to global best practices.

5. International Standards for Risk Management Plans (RMPs):
To be granted marketing authorization in certain regions, including the EU, MAHs must submit their applications for marketing authorization together with RMPs, which outline their plans for identifying, characterizing, and managing risks.

Indian Measures: While risk management plans are not legally mandated in India, it is expected that they would play a critical role in pharmacovigilance initiatives.

6. Periodic Safety Update Reports, or PSURs:

Global Conditions: In the EU, PSURs are a standard requirement for marketing authorization holders to provide updates about the safety profile of their products on a regular basis.

Indian Measures: India also requires PSURs to be filed in compliance with global pharmacovigilance criteria.

7. Global Requirements for Individual Case Safety Reports (ICSRs) Electronic Submission: Two of the numerous regions that have transitioned to electronic ICSR submission using standardized formats (like E2B) include the EU and the US.

Indian Measures: PvPI promotes electronic submission of ICSRs, although format variations may occur.

8. Local specifics and subtleties:

Global Conditions: Global norms give broad principles, but national laws may vary based on specific conditions in each region.

Indian Measures: India may have certain requirements when it comes to the oversight of clinical trials and post-marketing surveillance, for instance, pharmaceutical companies that have many sites need to be aware of these distinctions in order to stay in compliance with national and international pharmacovigilance laws, the regulatory bodies in each nation must provide regular updates so that one is aware of any changes or additions to the pharmacovigilance laws.

Question Set
PART-I

1. Describe the history and development of Pharmacovigilance.
2. Define PvPI? Write in details about the PvPI in India.
3. Describe the safety Monitoring of Medicines
4. State the importance of safety monitoring of medicines with that write full forms of CDER and CTCAE?
5. Write down the importance of safety monitoring of medicines and full form of CTCAE.
6. Define and classify ADR
7. Describe about the management of ADR.
8. Describe ADR and any three terminologies used in Pharmacovigilance in detail
9. Describe Predictability assessment
10. Describe Reporting
11. Describe seriousness assessment
12. Describe specialized resources for ADRs
13. Describe the benefit-risk ratio in detail
14. Differentiate in detail in ADR And Side effects
15. Differentiate in detail in Observed and Historical ADR
16. Estimate the time used to document adverse drug reactions that may be removed from CPRS
17. State Reporting problems in detail
18. Write a note on post approval expedited reporting.
19. Describe any five regulatory terminologies in detail
20. Describe any five terminologies of adverse medication-related events
21. State detail about any five terminologies used in pharmacovigilance
22. Summarize the impact of polypharmacy.
23. Explain daily defined dose.
24. Write in detail about the International Classification of Disease
25. Distinguish the WHO drug dictionaries
26. Explain MedDRA and its standard queries.
27. State detail about international Nonproprietary names for drugs
28. Define the basic information resources in pharmacovigilance?
29. Estimate the basic drug information resources
30. Explain drug databases
31. State detail about Eudra-vigilance
32. State the summary of Product Characteristics in detail
33. Explain CRO's and the importance of CRO's in the national program
34. Explain the impact of pharmacovigilance in hospitals.
35. Explain in detail about Vaccine Pharmacovigilance
36. Write various observational methods for vaccine safety study.

37. Describe Cross sectional studies and Case control studies.

38. Explain in detail about cohort studies and targeted clinical investigations

39. Explain in detail about stimulated reporting

40. Explain in detail the case-control study and cohort study

41. Explain in detail about communication in drug safety crisis management

42. Explain in detail about communication with regulatory agencies and media

43. Explain the importance of communication in drug safety crisis management.

44. State the importance of communication with Regulatory agencies and Business partners.

45. Write the importance of communication in pharmacovigilance.

46. Distinguish between Inclusion and Exclusion Criteria

47. Describe Serious Adverse Event

48. Discuss the requirements of ICSR.

49. Explain about post approval expedited reporting.

50. Explain the data should be reported in expedited reporting.

51. Explain the Investigator's responsibility in GCP.

52. Identify the Sponsors responsibility and ADR reporting guideline in GCP

53. Summarize the planning of pharmacovigilance.

54. Record drug safety evaluation in pediatrics.

55. Record drug safety evaluation in pregnancy and lactation.

56. Write down about CIOMS form.

57. Estimate the requirements in Indian and global pharmacovigilance.

58. Express the detail submission process of CDSCO reporting form.

59. Represent schedule Y in detail.

60. Sketch the functions of CDSCO.

Question Set
PART-II

1. Describe the safety monitoring of medicines
2. Discuss the history and development of Pharmacovigilance.
3. Explain how to establish a national program in Pharmacovigilance
4. Compare ADR and ADE
5. Compare detection and reporting
6. Compare Predictability and Causality assessment
7. Compare Reporting and Detection
8. Compare Severity and Seriousness assessment with example.
9. Describe detection in pharmacovigilance
10. Describe management of Adverse drug reaction
11. Describe predictability assessment in detail
12. Describe predictability, preventability and management of ADR.
13. Describe Preventability assessment in detail
14. Describe reporting and causality assessment
15. Describe Reporting and detection
16. Describe severity assessment in detail
17. Describe signal detection and data mining
18. Explain the process of reporting
19. Write a short note on methods in causality assessment.
20. Describe Adverse medication related event terminologies in pharmacovigilance
21. Define PvPI? Write in details about the PvPI in India.
22. Explain Medication Error
23. Describe the international classification of disease and daily defined dose.
24. Explain international classification of diseases
25. Explain therapeutical and chemical classification of drugs
26. Describe Drug Dictionaries and coding in pharmacovigilance
27. Explain in detail about MedDRA and Standardized MedDRA quarries
28. Explain the applications of MedDRA and standard MedDRA queries.
29. What are the different resources in pharmacovigilance and mentioned the different resources for ADR's?
30. Explain GCP in Pharmacovigilance studies.
31. Explain in detail about Contact Research Organization.
32. Explain the establishment procedure for pharmacovigilance in Hospitals
33. Write in detail about the CRO's
34. Explain in detail vaccine failure in pharmacovigilance
35. Explain in detail vaccine pharmacovigilance

36. What do you mean by vaccine pharmacovigilance and contrast various observational methods for vaccine safety study.

37. Compare and differentiate Active and passive surveillance

38. Compare Cross-sectional study and Cohort Study

39. Describe case control study and cohort study

40. Explain active and passive surveillance

41. Explain in detail about Drug Event Monitoring and registries

42. Give in details about Cross sectional studies and Case control studies.

43. Explain in detail about drug safety crisis management

44. Explain in detail about effect communication in pharmacovigilance

45. Explain the importance of communication in pharmacovigilance and does communication puts an impact on drug safety crisis management.

46. What is the importance of communication with regulatory agencies, business partners, Health care facilities and media?

47. Write the importance of communication in drug safety crisis management.

48. Explain in detail about premarketing clinical trials

49. Explain Pharmacovigilance well connected to clinical trials

50. Write in detail about the post marketing clinical trials

51. Describe ICSR in detail.

52. Explain in brief periodic safety update report.

53. Explain in detail about targeted clinical investigations

54. Organize the strategy to improve drug safety in pharmacovigilance

55. Summarize planning of pharmacovigilance in brief.

56. Write down about the drug safety evaluation in pregnancy and lactation

57. Write in detail on drug safety evaluation in pediatrics.

58. Write a short note on CIOMS working groups with their objectives.

59. Describe the role of DCGI and CDSCO

60. Explain in detail Schedule Y with the steps involved in it